Authentic Healing

A PRACTICAL GUIDE
FOR CAREGIVERS

Authentic Healing

A PRACTICAL GUIDE FOR CAREGIVERS

KATHI J. KEMPER, M.D., M.P.H.

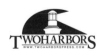
TWOHARBORS
WWW.TWOHARBORSPRESS.COM

Two Harbors Press
322 First Avenue N, 5th floor
Minneapolis, MN 55401
612.455.2293
www.TwoHarborsPress.com

ISBN-13: 978-1-63413-959-5
LCCN: 2015920572

Distributed by Itasca Books

Cover Design by Alan Pranke

Printed in the United States of America

Advance praise for *Authentic Healing*

"This is a must-read not only for physicians but for anyone who is a caregiver. You can feel Dr. Kemper's warmth exude throughout the pages as she describes physical, mental, and emotional preparations for healing as well as specific healing techniques. This book is timeless and will be a source of reference, encouragement, and inspiration for years to come."

JULIE MILUNIC
Publisher, *Natural Triad*

"*Authentic Healing* inspires both caregivers and clinicians. Dr. Kemper is a gifted healer who is also a recognized leader in integrative medicine and pediatrics."

DAVID RILEY, M.D.
Founder, Integrative Medicine Institute

"Dr. Kemper represents a new breed of physician who combines the best of conventional Western medicine with evidenced, informed holistic treatments. She gets to the heart of healing."

MIMI GUARNERI, M.D.
President, Academy Integrative Health and Medicine
Author, *The Heart Speaks: A Cardiologist Reveals the Secret Language of Healing*

"Dr. Kemper is bringing the most ancient of healing arts— spiritual healing—into the modern age. Doctors! Learn how to become a healer again and read this book! Patients! Give this book to your doctor!"

WAYNE JONAS, M.D.
President and CEO, Samueli Institute
Author, *Healing, Intention and Energy Medicine: Science, Research Methods and Clinical Implications*

"Dr. Kemper has done it again! This is a must-read for both doctors and patients. *Authentic Healing* allows the modern reader to tap into their physician-within by offering simple steps for spiritual, physical, and psychological healing. In the rapidly changing world of modern medicine, this book is a valuable tool for all those who seek to expand their knowledge of holistic and integrative medicine."

KATHLEEN O'KEEFE KANAVOS
Author, *Surviving Cancerland: Intuitive Aspects of Healing*

"Kathi Kemper is a medical doctor who understands healing—a healer who understands medicine: what a unique combination! This is a practical, warmhearted book on a complex subject; I am sure we will use it in our Therapeutic Touch classes."

MARTINE BUSCH,
Director, Van Praag Instituut
Netherlands

"Dr. Kemper has created a guide to mobilizing the body's life force through CHI (Compassionate Healing Intention) to access innate healing abilities. This book offers a valuable review of the scientific research on healing along with personal stories that illustrate the basic principles taught by skilled healers."

LARRY BURK, M.D.
Author, *Let Magic Happen: Adventures in Healing with a Holistic Radiologist*

"World-renowned pediatrician, Kathi J. Kemper M.D., M.P.H., builds on her indelible contribution to medicine by guiding us into the art of healing. Covering topics such as centering and grounding, preparing mentally and spiritually, and using intention and distance healing to help patients, and showcasing a plethora of techniques, Dr. Kemper offers ways to move beyond the 'diagnose and dispense model of care' into compassionate transmission of healing energy. She explains hands-on healing in an accessible, compelling way for peers and patients alike."

MICHAEL COHEN, J.D.
Author, *The Practice of Integrative Medicine* and *Healing at the Borderland of Medicine and Religion*

"Dr. Kemper is a visionary and pioneer in integrative medicine. Her work awakens us to the deeper aspects of healing within the mind, body, and spirit. She is a physician who believes in the attributes of the heart: those of practicing simple kindness, compassion, and gratitude, thus empowering others to participate in their own healing process and the maintenance of their health and/or well-being. Her life's work amplifies the strength and beauty that lies within, bringing inspiration to us all."

DEBORAH LARRIMORE, RN, BSN, LMBT, CHTP/I

"In *Authentic Healing*, Dr. Kathi Kemper again shows herself to be a masterful teacher, able to adroitly guide her students to new levels of insight and impact in patient care. She is a visionary leader in the art and science of healing, weaving ancient traditions and modern science to the enormous benefit of both patients and caregivers."

HILARY MCCLAFFERTY, M.D.
Director, Integrative Pediatric Residency, University of Arizona

"*Authentic Healing* reminds us that the art of healing is alive and well, and that the practice of medicine is far more than diagnosing disease and dispensing pills. This book is essential reading for anyone drawn to the healing professions."

DEAN RADIN, PH.D.
Author, *Supernormal: Science, Yoga, and the Evidence for Extraordinary Psychic Abilities*

"This book lovingly brings to us an understanding of healing which transcends time and space. It is not a medical book about curing diseases but about how a person can be healed as they activate their life force with love, no matter which healing modality they choose to use. It is really about how Dr. Kathi Kemper has lived her entire life bringing healing to herself and the world she lives in. Beautifully written and illustrated, it is a treasure."

GLADYS MCGAREY, M.D.
Founder, American Holistic Medical Association
Author, *Living Medicine: the Dwelling Place* and *The Physician Within You*

"Dr. Kemper is a true pioneer in a field that is slowly realizing that health is more about a process than a pill. She artfully brings the reader through a series of steps that helps prepare to skillfully recruit healing mechanisms. The most valued caregiver will be the one who can reproduce the teachings in this text. Dr. Kemper is a scholar, gifted teacher, and master clinician. This text should be required reading for anyone interested in using themselves as a healing vector."

DAVID RAKEL, M.D.
Author, *Integrative Medicine*

"*Authentic Healing* represents a turning point in the evolution of natural healing and the science of an integrative approach to care. Dr. Kemper has developed an excellent guide to understanding the value of the Ancient Art of Healing."

MARY JO RUGGIERI, PH.D.
Director, Institute for Holistic Health Careers

"*Authentic Healing* is a call to rediscover a lost art in medicine, from a time when being a physician meant practicing the art of healing in the deepest sense of the word—which is really about facilitating and supporting others in healing themselves. By combining the ancient arts of healing with the modern science of medicine, Dr. Kemper offers a vision of truly holistic and integrative health and wellness."

DZUNG VO, M.D.
Author, *The Mindful Teen: Powerful Skills to Help You Handle Stress One Moment at a Time*

"Fifteen percent of illnesses require drugs or surgery, and even those benefit from the skills of a skillful healer. The other 85% are far better healed with the wide array of alternatives presented by a real doctor who exemplifies the real healer archetype. Here is that legitimate wisdom."   .

C. NORMAN SHEALY, M.D., PH.D.
President and Professor Emeritus of Energy Medicine, Holos University Graduate Seminary
Past President, American Holistic Medical Association,
Author, *Living Bliss: Major Discoveries Along the Holistic Path*

"That such a brilliant and accomplished researcher and renowned medical doctor can make the sensitive and complex topic of 'healing' so sensible and accessible for all is just another example of the brilliance and insight of this prolific author. Science and spirituality are woven into compelling reading, ultimately offering a practical, do-it-yourself guide to inner peace. This, her fourth book, may be a key to more than healing ourselves, but to healing our families, communities, schools, and all of the helping and health professions. Thank you, Dr. Kemper, for opening this door not only to *Authentic Healing* but also to the authentic Kathi Kemper. This book will help heal our world."

REBECCA SHORE, PH.D.
Associate Professor of Educational Leadership, University of North Carolina at Charlotte
Author, *Baby Teacher: Nurturing Neural Networks from Birth to Age Five*

ALSO BY KATHI J. KEMPER, M.D., M.P.H.

*The Holistic Pediatrician: A Pediatrician's
Comprehensive Guide to Safe and Effective
Therapies for the 25 Most Common Ailments of
Infants, Children, and Adolescents*

Praise for *The Holistic Pediatrician:*

"The most important and comprehensive book you can read to
ensure the health of your child."

JOAN BORYSENKO, PH.D.
Author, *Minding the Body, Mending the Mind*

"A must-read for all pediatricians and the families they serve."

HENRY BERNSTEIN, D.O.
Chief of General Pediatrics, North Shore University Hospital

"Dr. Kemper fields the gamut of rumors from folk medicine to
cyberspace with equal aplomb. She has a wry sense of humor . . .
and a warmth that both inspires confidence and disarms."

The Seattle Times

"As the owner of a network of market-specific holistic health
magazines, I can't think of any book that I would recommend more
for parents who want to keep their children as healthy as possible . .
. naturally. *The Holistic Pediatrician* is comprehensive, incorporating
both mainstream and integrative therapies to help educate and aid
parents as they deal with common childhood health issues. Written
by a distinguished and highly respected pediatrician, this book
reflects both her compassion and her vast knowledge of traditional
and holistic medicine. With her definitive eye for detail, all

recommendations are evidence based with safety and effectiveness always at the forefront. Her warmth, caring, and desire for the wellness of our children shines through."

JULIE MILUNIC
Publisher, *Natural Triad*

Mental Health, Naturally

Winner of the 2011 Silver Award from Nautilus Books, the 2012 Gold Award from Forward Reviews, and the 2012 winner in the Body/Mind/Spirit Category Indie Book Award

Praise for *Mental Health, Naturally*

"Dr. Kemper is the new Dr. Spock of modern health care! Here is the best guide for keeping your children (and our future) both happy and healthy."

WAYNE JONAS, M.D.
President and Chief Executive Officer, Samueli Institute
Author, *Healing Intention and Energy Medicine: Science, Research Methods, and Clinical Implications*

"Insightful, sensitive, and evidence based. Dr. Kemper takes us on a truly healing journey."

MIMI GUARNERI, M.D., F.A.C.C.
Medical Director, Scripps Center for Integrative Medicine
The Heart Speaks

"Brilliant integration of modern science supporting the ancient wisdom: A Sound Mind in a Sound Body."

KENNETH PELLETIER, PH.D.
Author, *The Best Alternative Medicine*
Clinical Professor of Medicine, University of Arizona

"An authoritative, practical, and comprehensive guide. A must-read for anyone interested in cultivating a healthy mind in a healthy body."

AMIT SOOD, M.D., M.SC.
Author, *The Mayo Clinic Guide to Stress-Free Living*

"Beautifully written, heartfelt, compassionate, and scientifically precise, *Mental Health, Naturally* by Dr. Kathi Kemper is a must-read for anyone with an interest in or need for an integrative approach to mental health."

VICTOR SIERPINA, M.D.
WD and Laura Nell Nicholson Family Professor of Integrative Medicine
Professor, Family Medicine, University of Texas Medical Branch

"When you combine information with inspiration, some remarkable results can be achieved. *Mental Health, Naturally* can guide you and coach you to achieve the life you desire. Kemper's book can be your midwife to a new life."

BERNIE SIEGEL, M.D.
Author, *Faith, Hope, and Healing: Inspiring Lessons Learned from People Living with Cancer* and *Prescriptions for Living: Inspirational Lessons for a Joyous, Loving Life*

Addressing ADD Naturally

Praise for *Addressing ADD Naturally*

"A primer for parents who want to positively change their child's life. I cannot wait to give this book to my patients' parents."

CHRIS MAGRYTA, M.D., Pediatrician, Salisbury Pediatric Associates, NC

"This book is fantastic! It is written by a founding member of the field who is able to combine a wealth of knowledge with practical experience to offer effective guidance for a challenging condition. A must-read for any clinician or parent."

DAVID RAKEL, M.D.
Editor, *Integrative Medicine*
Family Physician, University of Wisconsin

"This short, sweet, practical book is comprehensive, evidence based, and gives step-by-step directions for successful change. It is helpful for the individual and the entire family. I love the big picture aspect as well as the individual."

PAULA GARDINER, M.D., M.P.H.
Family Medicine, Boston Medical Center

"In her book, Dr. Kathi Kemper gives us an excellent resource for parents who want to help their children improve their attention, focus, and self-discipline. She gives us detailed information for developing healthy habits and healthy environments for our children. A must-read."

ANNETTE FRANKS

"Finally! A book has been written by one of the best integrative pediatricians in the country. Dr. Kathi Kemper naturally addresses the ADD problem plaguing our schools and homes and supplies the reader with amazing information that does not depend solely on pharmaceuticals. Dr. Kemper has done the research and written the book we have all anxiously been awaiting. Too often society thinks that by drugging a problem, we've solved the bad behavior. Dr. Kemper's book, *Addressing ADD Naturally*, gives us other natural choices that work to generate health in the home, at play, and in the school system. Thank you, Dr. Kemper."

KATHLEEN O'KEEFE KANAVOS

This book is dedicated to all who aspire to bring comfort and relieve suffering, with deepest gratitude to my teachers: Dr. Norman Shealy, Dora Kunz, Susan Wager, Sandy Revesz, Jane Cornman, Dolores Krieger, Roy Bauer, Rosalyn Bruyere, Deborah Larrimore, and the many patients, friends, and colleagues who have allowed us to participate in their healing.

Acknowledgments

THERE ARE MANY PEOPLE TO THANK for helping this book become a reality, but first among them must be my dear friend, Julie Milunic, publisher of *Natural Triad*, who encouraged me to submit the first few chapters back in 2010. Thank you for your patience and encouragement. Thank you to Bob Parker, who called to encourage me to finish it. Thanks to Diane Habash for reading the first drafts with keen eyes, finding and gently identifying typographic errors and opportunities for greater clarity.

The book would not have been possible without my first introduction to Therapeutic Touch by Helen Bee. And as this student was ready, a series of extraordinary teachers and mentors appeared. Thank you to Dora Kunz, Dolores Krieger, Dr. Susan Wager, Sandy Revesz, and Jane Cornman for helping me begin to learn about Therapeutic Touch. I will always be grateful, and I will always remain a beginner humbly learning from your wise and insightful experience and compassion. Thank you to my dear friend, Martine Busch, whose tireless dedication has brought Therapeutic Touch to thousands of nurses and other health professionals across the Netherlands. Thanks to Diane May for her humorous, wise, and inspiring books on TT. Thanks to those who maintain Camp Indralaya and Pumpkin Hollow as sanctuaries for learning the sacred art of Therapeutic Touch.

Thanks to my dear nursing friends, Mary Jane Ott and Deborah Larrimore, for introducing me to Healing Touch and helping me learn by teaching others. Deborah, your courage in stepping into the unknown to teach Therapeutic Touch and Healing Touch to medical students marks you as a true pioneer. Thanks to Dr. Chuck Tegeler for bravely bringing HT to Wake Forest Baptist Health through translational research; to Suzanne Danhauer for her research on patients; and Rong Tang for leading the research on the effects of HT on the nurses who learn to provide it. Thanks to Tammy Shimfessel for being the Healing Touch nurse in our research on the interpersonal physiologic effects of compassion and to Hossam Shaltout for objectively measuring and analyzing the outcomes. Thanks to Dr. Caryl Guth for supporting the integration of ancient energy medicine into a modern academic medical center through her generous gift of an endowed Chair in Integrative Medicine, which it was my honor to occupy for five years.

Thanks to Roy Bauer, who insisted I learn about, become initiated in, and eventually become a Reiki master; Roy taught me about healing through his kind example in and outside the hospital and made me think about why doctors don't think of themselves as healers.

Thanks to Dr. David Steinhorn for his persistence in making sure I learned something about shamanism.

Thanks to the nursing organizations—the American Holistic Nurses Association, Nurse Healers Associates, and Therapeutic Touch International—who maintain such high standards for education and practice.

Thanks to the researchers, Marilyn Schlitz and Dean Radin, at the Institute for Noetic Sciences and to Rollin McCraty at the Institute of HeartMath, whose dedication to cutting-edge research gives us hope that we will someday understand the mechanisms of healing work as well as the fact that non-local healing is possible and does occur. Thanks to Dr. Wayne Jonas and his pioneering leadership at NIH and at the helm of the Samueli Institute for supporting and disseminating research on optimal healing environments and biofield healing. Thanks to Dr. Larry Dossey for his many inspiring books and articles on non-local healing and healing prayer.

Thanks to Dr. Herbert Benson for making me realize a career in medicine was possible for someone focused on meditation and mind–body health and to Dr. Gladys McGarey for encouraging me to apply.

Thank you to Dr. Norm Shealy for being a role model and mentor of an integrative physician—you remain twenty years ahead of your time.

Thanks to my wonderful North Carolina neighbors, the Messicks, for being the best friends and supporters wherever my work has taken me. Unending thanks to the patients, friends, and colleagues who have allowed me the great privilege of participating in their healing journeys.

And deepest thanks to Daniel, who makes it all worthwhile.

Contents

Introduction

AFTER MORE THAN THIRTY YEARS, I'm finally coming out of the closet. I've been to medical school, completed a residency and a fellowship, taught at prestigious medical schools, received NIH grants, conducted research, held leadership positions in national medical societies, and published more than 150 papers in peer-reviewed scientific journals. But now I'm coming out. I admit it. Although I graduated as a doctor and learned many useful skills, I really went to medical school to learn how to be a healer. I didn't. It's taken decades and guidance from some of the nation's best healers, but I've finally learned enough to write about what I wish I'd learned when I was that young medical student who wanted to know how to heal. I'm writing this for those who are like me, who want a basic introduction to healing from a reputable, reliable resource.

Back in the 1990s, I taught and conducted research at Harvard's Boston Children's Hospital. Another doctor asked for my help with a challenging patient. The patient was a teenage boy who was dying from a tumor despite several rounds of aggressive treatment. His father wanted a healer. I called Roy, the only man I could think of who might fit the bill. Roy was a former Catholic priest who had become a

1

shaman and Reiki healer. Roy came to the hospital with his drums, feathers, holy water, and prayers. Over two hours, he worked as the boy dozed, his father watched, and the hospital staff kept a curious, but respectful, distance. The father and boy grew more peaceful. When Roy finished, the boy awoke and told his father that he'd seen a white owl in his dreams. Somehow, everyone knew that the owl was a symbol that his time here was limited. Through his tear-filled eyes, the father thanked us for the healing. A few days later, the boy died.

This profound experience, set in a teaching hospital of one of the premiere academic institutions in the United States, raised several questions for me. What is the difference between healing and curing? Why, when the boy's father asked for a healer, did the hospital staff (including me), known nationally for their medical expertise, not offer themselves, but instead called someone else who had no formal biomedical training? Can doctors, nurses, other health professionals, and dedicated laypersons learn to heal, or is it simply a gift for the very few? Can healing be learned? What preparation is required? How do we get started? What else do we need to know?

This book is written to answer these questions to empower caregivers like you to become more effective healers. It's written in four parts that logically flow from one to another.

Part 1 answers basic questions:

- What is the difference between healing and curing?
- What are the basic requirements to become a healer?
- Who is the real healer?

- What do healers mean by "centering" and "grounding"?
- What are the different types of healing, and what is the evidence that they improve health?

Part 2 takes you on the first steps toward preparing to heal—physically, emotionally, mentally, and spiritually. You will learn and gain experience with basic breathing techniques to bring your intention, body, mind, and spirit into alignment. You will explore basic anatomy from both a modern biomedical perspective and from ancient healing traditions like Ayurveda and Traditional Chinese Medicine. Part 2 provides a solid foundation for starting your healing practice.

Part 3 gives you a step-by-step guide to the most commonly used healing strategies and practices and provides you with exercises to help you gain confidence. We will start with simple warm-up practices, and then move to techniques to help you calm and relax another person who is feeling stressed or tense. You will also learn techniques to help energize and restore vitality for someone who feels fatigued or wiped out. Helping reduce pain is another important goal, and you will learn how to more effectively comfort someone who is hurting. Step-by-step instructions are also provided on how to soothe swelling (edema) and bloating, nausea, and constipation. Finally, you will learn how to effectively work with a partner on behalf of a recipient—whether the partner is a health professional, family member, or pastoral care worker.

Part 4 explores related ideas like distance (non-local) healing, what kinds of advice or homework you can give to help recipients continue to benefit between healing sessions, and answers to trainees' most frequently asked questions.

After considering several options about how to handle

references (I am an academic physician, after all, and there is plenty of scientific evidence to support healing as an evidence-based practice), I've decided to include references as footnotes. This makes it easy for you to find original research without having to flip to the back of the book. If you don't want to read the footnotes, you don't have to, but when you share this book with skeptics, you'll be glad the references are there.

Ready to dive in? Let's start by answering basic questions in Part 1.

PART 1

Basic Questions

CHAPTER 1
Beginner's Mind

REGARDLESS OF OUR TRAINING, we all start on the path of healing as beginners. Beginners' questions are often the most profound questions, the ones we continue to reflect on the longer and deeper our practice becomes.

1. What Is the Difference between Healing and Curing?

Curing is one of the main goals of modern medicine (the others being prevention, management, and rehabilitation). Curing refers to a disease. We cure strep throat with penicillin. Many cancers can be cured with chemotherapy or radiation therapy. Cataracts can be cured with surgery. There is no cure (yet) for the common cold or for many chronic health problems like diabetes, depression, and osteo-arthritis, but many are managed with chronic use of medications, canes, or crutches, and a healthier lifestyle.

Healing refers to restoring a sense of health, vitality, or well-being. Healing refers to the whole person, and restoring a sense of order, orga-nization, integrity, balance, ease, or harmony to a dynamic whole. The person who is ill, injured, or suffering is the one who does the healing. A doctor places a cast, but the injured person heals the broken bone.

"Nature alone cures . . . and what nursing has to do . . . is to put the patient in the best condition for Nature to act upon him."

—FLORENCE NIGHTINGALE

Someone who heals despite a serious illness or injury is a good healer. So, if you have survived cancer, a heart attack, or injuries from a car crash, you are a good healer.

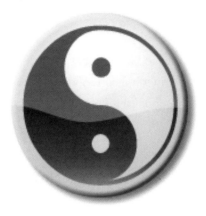

Yin and Yang of Curing and Healing

In Asian medicine, yin and yang are the opposites that are both necessary for the whole. Yin is inner, quiet, subtle, and dark; yang is outer, loud, obvious, and bright. Yin is healing; yang is curing. Yin is for people. Yang addresses disease. In the greatest yin, there is some yang. In the greatest yang, there is also some yin.

Yin (healing) treatment > Person > Person feels better > Better specific health outcomes

Yang (curing) treatment > Disease > Better specific health outcomes > Person feels better

Can a Dying Person Be Healed?

All things change. Atoms and molecules are in motion. Stars arise and flame out. Everything that is born eventually dies, from the smallest flower to the largest whale. Human bodies die, too, of course. Nevertheless, people can die with a sense of peace, purpose, harmony, comfort, and connectedness to others. In this way, they can be said to be healed, even though their bodies die.

2. Can Other People Heal the Sick?

The answer is a paradox—both yes and no. Let's think about it by analogy. Can a comedian make you laugh? Truthfully, it's hard to *force* someone to laugh, but comedians can certainly *help* us laugh. Great actors can "make" us cry, surprise us, disgust us, frighten us, and help us feel all kinds of emotions. Their ability to engender those emotions in others is what makes them great entertainers.

Parents, teachers, and others also offer insight into the question of whether we can heal. Calm parents soothe crying children. They do not *make* their children feel better, but they create an atmosphere of calm reassurance that promotes a child's confidence and sense of security. Skillful teachers help their students master material they thought they'd never understand. Sincere prayer offered by a devout spiritual leader can inspire hope and facilitate a sense of meaning to life's hardships. Skilled mediators facilitate understanding and forgiveness between people in conflict. So, yes! Common sense and our own experience confirms that just as doctors place stitches to facilitate physical healing; just as parents promote emotional well-being; just as teachers support students to master mentally challenging material; just as spiritual leaders foster hope; and just as mediators encourage social harmony, so it is possible for people to facilitate another individual's healing on many different levels. But we cannot *make* another person healed or whole.

3. What Are the Basic Requirements for Being a Healer?

There are a few simple requirements for becoming a healer:

- Compassion: the desire to relieve suffering
- Good health: physical, emotional, mental, and spiritual vitality; being cheerful, resilient, calm, and peaceful
- Focus: the ability to direct attention for a sustained period of time
- Dedication and discipline: the willingness and ability to practice, to learn, and to grow
- Openness and flexibility: curiosity about participating in healing rather being dogmatic about the method or outcome
- Non-judgmental acceptance: willingness to accept things that arise and unexpected outcomes as they are
- Collaborative, empowering attitude: working in respectful partnership with the person seeking help, not attempting to dominate or control the person or the outcome
- Detachment and humility: while maintaining compassion, the healer remains detached from the specific results and does not claim credit for the results, knowing that ultimately, healing is up to the person seeking help, nature, and the environment in which the person lives

We'll talk more about these basic requirements in subsequent chapters. For now, consider the practice of healing to be similar to learning a new sport or musical instrument. It takes practice as well as good coaching to master a new skill.

4. Is Everyone Who Claims to Be a Healer Really a Healer?

No, I'm sad to say. Although most people have a sincere desire to help others, sometimes people are driven by pride, greed, the desire to dominate others, or a craving for fame; hatred, envy, or skepticism about conventional medications; or the need to overcome their own wounds rather than compassion. If someone who claims to be a healer jumps right in and starts to work on you without asking your permission, decline the offer; he is working from his need, not yours. If someone who claims to be a healer demands that you undress (outside of a medical exam setting); insists that you adopt his belief system or religion; makes outrageous claims (I can cure cancer or heal your stroke, diabetes, multiple sclerosis, etc.); or otherwise makes you uncomfortable, politely but firmly decline. While spontaneous healing is possible with any condition, true healers never claim credit for the results and are humbly empowering, not dominating.

5. Why Don't Health Professionals Call Themselves Healers?

Health professionals dedicate their working lives to preventing and relieving suffering. Hospitals are built to cure the sick. But few of us who work in hospitals consider ourselves healers. Why is that?

Before we had powerful medications and surgery, medicine had very few treatments that actually cured diseases. As our ability to prevent, cure, and manage serious, life-threatening diseases grew (for example, to prevent smallpox, polio, typhoid, measles, cholera, and rheumatic fever; cure tuberculosis, syphilis, scarlet fever, and some kinds of cancer; and manage diabetes, kidney failure, heart disease, HIV, and near-sightedness), we focused more on the medicines and the diseases and less on the people involved. And as health care has become more expensive and as the insurance and pharmaceutical industries have grown more powerful, we have focused the lens of our attention and effort almost entirely on diagnoses and treatments—the "diagnose and dispense" model of care.

My good friend, Sam, who retired after many years as a successful businessman, often said to me, "Tell me what you get paid to do, and I'll tell you what you do." These days, doctors, clinics, and hospitals get paid for making diagnoses and providing treatments promoted by pharmaceutical companies and approved by insurance companies. There may be plenty of scientific evidence that another treatment would be beneficial, but unless that treatment is covered by insurance, it is unlikely that you will hear about it from your doctor. There is no DSM[1] diagnosis, no CPT[2] code, no ICD-9[3] code, and no DRG[4] related to healing. Consciously engaging in healing, offering sincere goodwill, wise insight, or encouragement and inspiring hope may be important, but they are not directly reimbursable and do not generate profits for pharmaceutical and device manufacturers or the medical management sector[5], so you will not see ads for them.

---

1 DSM, Diagnostic and Statistical Manual of Mental Disorders
2 CPT, Current Procedural Terminology which describes medical and surgical interventions
3 ICD-9 is the ninth official version of the International Statistical Classification of Diseases and Health-related Problems
4 Diagnosis-Related Group, a classification system for biomedical diagnoses
5 Some people refer to the medical management sector as the U.S. health system, but because it's not a system in the sense of a deliberately created national system designed to promote health, but instead has arisen in the context of a set of interrelated business and professional enterprises, I refer to it in its economic sense as a sector of the economy.

6. Does Healing Work? And If So, How?

Yes. Diagnoses, cures, and treatments are external and objective. Healing is internal, personal, and subjective. Knowing whether or not a bone has knit, a tumor has shrunk, or a kidney is working is pretty straightforward using modern technology. Knowing whether someone feels more at peace, has a greater sense of harmony, comfort, confidence, connection, or well-being is much more difficult. It requires introspection, self-awareness, and communication. Nevertheless, based on vast human experience and an increasing number of scientific studies, we can conclude that healing happens. Most often, people notice that they feel calmer, more peaceful, relaxed, trusting, and have less anxiety, stress, and discomfort.

How Does Healing Happen?

Mainstream medical science is based on the laws of Newtonian physics, chemistry, and biology. Increasingly, medicine understands the importance of psychological and social sciences, too. Modern social psychology informs us that we exert enormous influence on one another, even, and perhaps most powerfully, when we're not consciously aware of it.

Healing (particularly in-person, hands-on healing) can be understood, at least in part, as a benefit of positive interpersonal dynamics. Spending time with someone who is calm, encouraging, cheerful, and interested in our well-being is uplifting. It helps us relax and feel hopeful. Those emotions can slow the cascade of stress hormones that impede healing, and they bolster the release of neuro-hormones that promote greater comfort and vitality.

Consider this analogy. If someone is humming a variety of notes absentmindedly, in no particular order or rhythm, and another person

13

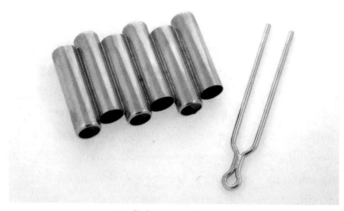

©Maljalen – Fotolia.com

comes along who sings a very clear note or tune, the hummer soon joins in. It's almost impossible to continue to hum something else when a powerful, skilled singer starts singing. In an orchestra, just one instrument sounds the keynote with a tuning fork, pitch pipe or instrument, and everyone else attunes to that tone.

Similarly, most of the time, and especially when we are ill, our "singing" is scattered by worry, pain, and distress. When someone else is able to hold a strong sense of clear, calm compassion and confidence, the scattered senses and attitudes begin to align with that. You might call this *interpersonal resonance*[6].

Even skeptics would agree that this kind of interaction offers at least a powerful placebo effect. The placebo effect is a physiologic modulator of psycho-neuro-immunologic systems, but it is usually considered less powerful than "real" medications.

---

6 We'll talk more about resonance in Chapter 2 when we discuss the importance of the healer being centered and grounded. Briefly, if the healer isn't centered and grounded, she can start resonating with the patient, unconsciously adopting the patient's pain and becoming more scattered and distressed, leading to burnout and ineffectiveness.

7. Is Healing Just a Placebo?

First of all, activating the internal psycho-neuro-immunologic systems through a placebo is very powerful! Placebos engage the body's innate healing systems and are so effective that modern scientists have to work very hard to make sure that the improvements we see with "new and improved" medications are not driven by the powerful placebo effect.

Second, I believe that healing is even more than a placebo treatment. Based on emerging research and my experience offering healing to infants, animals, plants, and comatose patients who are generally not susceptible to placebo effects, it looks like something beyond the placebo effect or patients' expectations or hopes is at work.

8. Is Healing Due to an Electromagnetic Energy?

Maybe. Recent research on biological electromagnetic fields has shown that the field generated by our heart (the signals detected on an ECG) extends several feet beyond our body. In fact, the electrical signals from one person's heart can be detected in the brain waves of a person nearby[7]. Are the subtle variations in electromagnetic signals generated by the healer somehow influencing the field of the recipient in a way that promotes healing? This would be a fascinating arena for research.

Is healing based on some kind of pattern or information transmitted from one person to another? Another great research question! Quantum physics informs us that the human element (consciousness) affects reality, not just our perception of reality. Does healing happen

---

7 McCraty R., et al., "The electricity of touch: Detection and measurement of cardiac energy exchange between people," in K.H. Pribram, editor. Brain and Values: Is a Biological Science of Values Possible. (Mahwah: Lawrence Erlbaum Associates, 1998), 359–379.

on a quantum level? I don't know. Is healing based on a subtle energy, vital energy, or etheric fields? I don't know, and as a scientist, I don't even know how to test those theories. Because most ancient healing practices are based on a belief in some kind of vital energy or universal life energy, and because many healers describe the process in terms of energy, I often use the term, too, even though it is not the same kind of energy we measure in high school physics or chemistry labs.

As a practical clinician, I believe that because healing is safe (if a few common-sense guidelines are followed), does not interfere with any mainstream medical treatment, and helps people, we don't need to know how it works to learn to use it. On the other hand, I plan to continue to do research in this field because I believe that through rigorous research, we can become better healers, fine-tuning our skills and our application of those skills.

9. Do You Have to Be Religious to Be an Effective Healer?

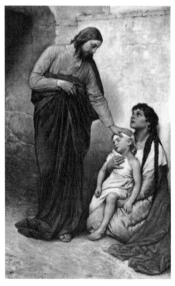

No. Jesus Christ is known as The Great Healer or The Master Healer. His disciples gained countless converts in part through their healing work. Many modern healers still heal in the name of Jesus. Dora Kunz developed the healing technique of Therapeutic Touch (now practiced by over 80,000 nurses internationally), in part by watching the Christian evangelist and faith healer, Kathryn

Gabriel von Max : *Jesus Heilt die Kranken*

Kuhlman. On the other hand, Christianity does not have a monopoly on healing. Great spiritual leaders from Islam, Hinduism, and Buddhism, as well as indigenous shamans, have also been acclaimed as healers. I am not aware of any effective healer who denies the importance of spirituality. But one does not need to be religious to be spiritual.

Regardless of religious background (or lack thereof), healing is a spiritual activity. It is intimate. It is sacred. It is meaningful. It calls on us to be present to something beyond our ordinary, limited sense of ourselves, and it affirms our connection with one another and something greater than our individual selves.

10. Can Healing Be Learned or Is It a Gift?

Yes! Healing is a gift and it can be learned. Just as a few people are naturally gifted musicians while others struggle to learn chopsticks, some people are naturally gifted at facilitating healing. And just as gifted athletes practice the fundamentals of their skills, those who want to learn how to help heal others need to practice, practice, practice. (Note: for simplicity, we will call those who facilitate, support, promote, encourage, and set the stage for healing *healers*. Please remember that this is just for simplicity. In reality, the person who achieves greater well-being is the healer.) Learning a new skill of any kind is easiest with good coaching, practice, feedback, and more practice. With dedication, good training, and persistence, even those who are not born healers can help reduce suffering.

Disclaimer

My dad was a basketball coach, and I've had some pretty good training. Still, I'm just five feet six. Even if I practiced for hours every day for the next ten years, I'd never be able to dunk a basketball like Michael Jordan or handle the ball like Chris Paul.

Likewise, when it comes to healing, I've had some of the world's best teachers and role models, and I've practiced many hours over many years. But I do not claim to be a superstar of the healing world. In important ways, this makes me a better teacher. Why?

I do not see auras. I do not hear voices telling me where to place my hands. I do not claim that ancient entities or animal spirits guide me. It took me two years of diligent practice just to begin to sense what I perceive as the human energy field with my hands. I learned the rudiments of using an ophthalmoscope and stethoscope much more quickly! And most of those I have taught these skills have learned them far more quickly than I did.

I am deeply grateful for CT scanners, MRIs, ultrasounds, EEGs, ECGs, and other tests to make an accurate assessment. At the same time, I know that learning and practicing healing has improved my intuition and made me a better clinician. Although I appreciate antibiotics, anesthetics, surgery, and other modern treatments, I'm grateful to have learned healing skills that help my patients feel more relaxed, revitalized, and comfortable.

How Does This Help You?

Because it's been challenging for me, I can anticipate your questions, your skepticism, and your self-doubt. I will focus on the fundamentals, not carry you off into fantasy land. If I saw auras like Dora Kunz or Rosalyn Bruyere, you might wonder if people who couldn't see auras can learn to help heal. If I saw spirit guides or had higher sensory perception like Barbara Brennan or Donna Eden, you might wonder if you had to have that kind of perception before you could start. I am here to tell you that even if your senses are limited to regular hearing, smell, taste, and touch, and you need glasses to read road signs, you can still learn to heal. I've been there. I've learned, and you can, too.

What's Next?

Next we'll explore the reasons for healing and find out if you're ready to start. Then we'll cover some physical, mental, and spiritual exercises to build your healing capacity. Just as practicing free throws, lay-ups, scales, and chords is not quite the same as playing a sport or music, they are very useful fundamentals to have under your belt when you are faced with the real thing. After you feel comfortable with the fundamentals, we move into learning some simple techniques you can use to help heal others and yourself. Ready to get started? Let's reflect on our basic motivation for doing healing work.

CHAPTER 2

Why Heal?
Who Are Healers?

ANY REPORTER WORTH HIS INK knows that a story answers the basic Ws: Why, Who, What, When, Where, and hoW. Before we dive into techniques and skills of healing, let's explore the fundamentals of Why and Who heals?

> "It concerns us to know the purposes we seek in life,
> For then, like archers aiming at a definite mark,
> We shall be more likely to attain what we desire."
>
> —ARISTOTLE

Consider the story about the three bricklayers, working side by side. When asked why they were laying brick, the first one answered, "I'm following the foreman's instructions." The second said, "I'm feeding my family." The third responded, "I'm building a cathedral." None of these answers is wrong, but when things get challenging (as they eventually do), some reasons inspire more persistence and dedication than others.

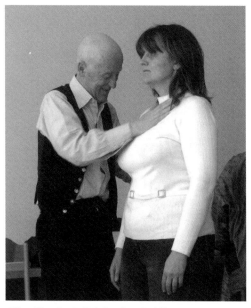

Clive Harris, Polish healer, Public Access, Wikimedia commons

Why do *you* want to be a healer[8]?

What motivates you to pursue this work?

What is your intention?

Reflect for a moment or two. Imagine you are entering a healing school. In fact, you have entered the healing school of life itself. Life's healing school has many courses and teachers (some of whom wear distressing disguises, as Mother Teresa observed). And each course offers an open-book, collaborative, self-graded exam that promotes your eventual mastery.

---

8 Remember that in reality a healer is someone who recovers from an illness, injury, or other health challenge. Here, however, we will use the term healer to refer to someone who assists in or facilitates the healing process.

The first lesson of the first course is to know yourself. As Dr. Dolores Krieger, co-founder of Therapeutic Touch has said, healers must be "more than masters of technique; they must be masters of themselves."[9] To master yourself, you must know yourself.

Know Yourself

> *"This above all, to thine own self be true.*
> *And it must follow, as the night the day,*
> *Thou canst not then be false to any man."*
>
> —WILLIAM SHAKESPEARE, *HAMLET*

The first open-book exam in the "know yourself" class has just three questions. Remember, there are no right or wrong answers, and you are not being graded.

Question 1. Why Do You Want to Be a Healer?

Aspirants to the health professions are asked: Why do you want to be a doctor? A nurse? An acupuncturist? Massage therapist? A physical therapist? Psychologist? Social worker? Pharmacist? Dietitian? Chiropractor?

Does one or more of these reasons resonate with you?

"I want to be a healer (or a healing presence, catalyst, channel, expediter, or facilitator, etc.) because:

- "I want to help other people."
- "I want to relieve suffering."
- "I want to better understand myself and others."
- "I want to understand the impact of human caring on health."

---

9 Krieger D., Therapeutic Touch: Inner Workbook, (Bear and Company, 1997)...

23

- "I want to be like my mom, dad, grandparent, uncle, or aunt, or the doctor who saved me or my loved one, or the nurse who comforted me in the emergency room, etc."
- "I want to be respected in my community, family, state, or nation."
- "I want to be able to take care of myself, my family, and my friends when we become ill or need help."
- "I want a steady paycheck to support my family."
- "I want to be someone's hero."
- "I want to be part of a dedicated team that serves humanity."
- "I want to be part of a noble profession or an enduring tradition."
- "I want to save lives."
- "I want to discover the cure for cancer, diabetes, multiple sclerosis, etc."
- "I want to make the world a better, more beautiful, peaceful, harmonious place."
- "I want to be more connected with other people."
- "I want to recognize, evoke, and celebrate the highest and best within myself and others."
- "I want to perceive, support, express, or evoke more beauty and harmony."
- "I want to transform health care to make it more humane and compassionate."
- "I want to use my God-given talents."
- "I want to follow my personal calling. "
- "It makes me feel good inside; it gives me a sense of pride; it makes my life meaningful."
- "I want to learn new things and test my limits."
- "I can't imagine doing anything else."

- "I want to become enlightened, to understand myself in relationship to the universe and other people."

Some people are satisfied with the first reason or two, "I want to help others," and "I want to relieve suffering," while others identify with several statements on this list. Very few people aim for the very last reason (attaining enlightenment), but it's okay to think out of the box. You may have another reason that's not even listed here. Remember, there is no right or wrong reason, and you are not being graded. This is an exam to help you know yourself.

If you identified more than one reason, it's time to narrow your list. Pick ONE that is the main reason YOU want to be a healer. Writing or telling someone strengthens your motivation and keeps you honest, so either write down your answer or tell another person. If you tell another person, please work with someone who will listen with an open mind and an attitude of curiosity and acceptance. You can take turns telling and listening, or you can just jot down your reason privately.

Let's repeat the process two more times. Each time we will ask WHY do you want to do THAT? Or WHY is THAT important to you? For example, you may have answered, "I want to help other people." The next step is to ask yourself, "Why do I want to help other people?" We ask the same questions to help you dive deeper into your own motivations and help you know yourself better.

Question 2. Why Do You Want to Do THAT (e.g., Help Others)? Why Is that Important to You?

Occasionally people resist this question, thinking the answer is obvious. Of course you want to help others. That's a good thing in and of itself. If you find yourself resisting question 2, take a breath. Relax. By taking one more step, you may surprise yourself. You might have just one or even several reasons you hadn't really noticed earlier. Here are some examples:

Why help others?

- To decrease suffering in the world.
- I feel uncomfortable when others suffer, so by helping others, I decrease my own suffering.
- So I can live in a world where people help each other.
- Because I believe in the Golden Rule. If I want to be helped, I should help others.
- Because that's how I was raised. Those are my family values.
- To fulfill others' expectations of me.
- So people will respect me, pay me, listen to me, or obey me.
- Because I feel more powerful when I can help someone else.
- Because I feel useful and valuable when others are grateful to me.
- To increase the sense of joy, trust, connection, vitality, or peace in the world one person at a time.
- To give my life meaning and purpose.
- To relieve boredom.
- To heal myself; to better know my inner self.
- To develop my talents, my intuitive skills.
- To answer an inner calling.
- To face and overcome my self-serving ego, my fears, and my small-mindedness.
- To transform my awareness.

- To decrease the need for treatments that are expensive or that have serious side effects.
- To be more connected to others, God, Nature, Spirit, or the life force.
- To experience and express compassion and loving-kindness.
- To feel the energy or power of Nature/God/Spirit move through me.
- To fully express my religious, philosophical, ethical, or spiritual beliefs.

You may like or dislike any of these reasons. You may have other reasons. There is no right or wrong answer to this question. There is simply greater self-understanding. Maintain an attitude of open-minded curiosity and non-judgmental acceptance. Before taking the next step, just jot down your answer(s) or tell it to someone you trust. Pick the ONE reason that is most important to you in this moment.

Question 3: Why Is THAT Reason Important to You?

As you move deeper into understanding your own motivation, you may find yourself at a loss for words. If so, feel free to explore this question with images, sounds, or movements. Sketch a picture; sense a color; recall a song or hum a tune; dance or move. You may sense a place in Nature or imagine a wise guide or inspirational person you are trying to emulate. You may remember a bit of poetry. If you prefer to explore this question in words, think out loud with a trusted, non-judgmental companion who will listen as you dive deep into your own motivations and re-emerge to express them. Or write a free-flowing stream of consciousness of words or ideas in a journal. You do not have to use complete sentences or correct grammar. You are getting to know yourself. Use the tools and techniques that fit you.

Exploring the question of "Why become a healer?" three times may seem excessive, but for many people, it brings a new sense of clarity and a stronger sense of purpose, meaning, and dedication. Hearing others' reasons can also strengthen your respect for them and your desire for them to succeed as you work toward common goals. This builds a sense of teamwork and collaboration, and decreases stress.

Congratulations! You have just completed an open-book exam. Did your answers surprise you? Before we take the next step together in learning to heal, let's establish three basic assumptions about who healers are. Being clear and explicit about assumptions helps us establish common ground.

Three Assumptions: Healers Are Humans Who:

1. Recognize, respect, and address their own personal needs skillfully in order to work collaboratively and respectfully with those who seek help to achieve health goals (patients or clients).
2. Avoid thoughts, words, and actions that increase suffering.
3. Offer peace, goodwill, kindness, and actions that facilitate the recipient's healing, but do not claim credit and are not attached to a particular outcome.

Assumption 1. Healers recognize, respect, and address their own personal needs skillfully in order to work collaboratively and respectfully with those who seek help to achieve health goals (patients or clients).

We are most effective when we are ready, willing, and able to help. In the real world, human beings are sometimes exhausted, hungry, thirsty, uncomfortable, confused, forgetful, sad, angry, or afraid. Sometimes the needs of our body, emotions, family, friends, and colleagues distract us from attending to others. Unless we honestly admit that we are human beings who also have legitimate needs and obligations, we may resort to unskillful strategies that jeopardize our effectiveness.

When we do not address our own needs effectively, it is tempting to view others' requests as burdens. This can result in unprofessional behavior, such as referring to patients as "hits" (those admitted from the emergency room to the hospital), "gomers" (those with complex, chronic needs who seek emergency care), or "crocks" (those whose emotional and mental distress manifests as physical pain or other symptoms). It can also dull our perception of another's request (e.g., delays in responding to "help" buttons, alarms, or messages). Unmet needs can also impair our focus and clarity, resulting in errors or poor quality of care.

An empty cup cannot pour.

Let's assume that when we work as healers, we are truly ready and able to help others with respect and compassion, not seeking to use them to meet our own basic needs or exploit them for our own wealth, power, or fame. Healers don't rely on those seeking help for emotional nurturing, sexual gratification, entertainment, or a sense of superiority. Healers do not disparage, bully, manipulate, or intimidate those asking for help. Healers do not perceive those seeking help as enemies or burdens, but as respected allies who provide us with the opportunity to do the work we really want to do.

Assumption 2. *Healers avoid thoughts, words, and actions that increase suffering.*

"First, do no harm" is a basic rule in the health professions. Healers do not diminish the person seeking help. Healers do not make someone feel worse than he already does. Healers do not "blame the victim" or ask why this person "did this to yourself," but offer comfort, safety, and companionship on the healing journey.

First, do no harm.

After establishing a sense of trust, safety, and shared intention, healers empower their patients, offering support without taking away dignity or free will. Healers are honest, discreet, and trustworthy. Healers use common sense, such as the basic hygiene of washing hands between clients to avoid carrying infections from one person to another.

Healers are hopeful yet humble. Healers do not raise false expectations through extravagant claims (e.g., this technique cures cancer, reverses aging, defeats diabetes, restores youthful vigor). Healers reassure patients that they can feel more relaxed, peaceful, and harmonious—the very conditions in which healing is most likely to occur.

Assumption 3. *Healers offer peace, goodwill, warm-heartedness, kindness, and actions that facilitate the recipient's healing, but do not claim credit and are not attached to a particular outcome.*

This is the first paradox of healing. Healers do not heal. Healers convey energy and information that patients can use to facilitate their own healing. We offer our highest intentions and our most thoughtful, informed, skillful actions, arranging an optimal environment for healing to occur, but in the final analysis, we do not MAKE anyone better. Patients heal themselves. Spiritual traditions often attribute healing to God, angels, Nature, or other spiritual forces. The patient accepts life energy and information from a spiritual realm to achieve a physical benefit. The healer may serve as a channel, a vessel, a conduit, or transmitter for these spiritual forces, but healing energy and information flow *through* (not *from*) the healer.

We may share a map, offer a cool drink, a brief respite, or walk with someone, but we do not take the journey for him. Coaches can help athletes improve their performance, but they do not run the race or play the concert for them. Embracing this paradox helps us avoid the traps of pride and attachment to specific outcomes, allowing us to remain more open, accepting, and flexible.

Humility

Dora Kunz, a well-known 20th-century healer who was a co-founder of the healing practice of Therapeutic Touch, would only claim that most of her patients would feel a bit more relaxed, comfortable, and hopeful. She was practical, humble, and refused to offer false hope or make outrageous claims. In Dora's words:

When I do healing, I try to be still and to have a sense of nonattachment to the results; I will do the best that I can for the person in need, meanwhile fully recognizing that the results—good or bad—are not totally in my hands. Even though we always want to be successful, we cannot be, because no person's destiny is fully in our hands.[10]

---

10 Dora Kunz with Dolores Krieger, The Spiritual Dimension of Healing Touch, (Rochester: Bear and Company, 2004), 165.

Next—What Do Healers Do?

We've established that you have strong, deep reasons for wanting to serve as a healer. We've also established that healers are humans who respect themselves and others, avoid increasing suffering, and extend acceptance and compassion, but do not take credit for the outcome. So, what do healers do? That's what the next chapter is all about.

CHAPTER 3

What Do Healers Do? What Are Centering and Grounding?

HAVING THE CLEAR INTENTION to be helpful to another person, to connect with him, and to relieve his suffering is essential for healing. This is the reason Chapter 1 was devoted to intention and motivation. An explicit intention and a strong motivation to help are *essential*, but they are not *sufficient* to create the conditions for healing to occur. Health professionals study for many years to master knowledge and skills to provide scientific medical care. The secret of the art of healing is knowing how to *be* as well as how to *do*. To become an effective healer, the two central practices are learning to become and remain *centered* and *grounded* while engaging in healing work. Regardless of whether the healer is trying to help someone relax, feel more energized, relieve pain, nausea, or some other symptom, or support a sense of peace, harmony, and ease, the healer practices centering and grounding.

What Are "Centering" and "Grounding"?

Centering

Centering is the core activity of the art of healing. Centering refers to the process of going within, withdrawing attention from the outer world of sensations, and even the inner activities of thoughts, worries, and emotions, to become consciously aware of and focused upon the peace, quiet, and harmony of the inner self. This deep inner self is also connected with the harmonious order of the universe.

Centering Sounds Like Meditation. Is It?

Yes. Centering is a form of meditation, an effortless effort. For most Americans, withdrawing attention to a quiet inner state is an unusual activity that requires a novel effort. Some may wonder if, in fact, there is any stillness within. You are wiser than you know. Without consciously thinking about it, your body is regulating your blood sugar levels, digestion, and metabolism; your immune system recognizes your own cells and protects them against foreign invaders in your skin, mouth, eyes, and digestive track without your conscious awareness; your kidneys cleanse your blood; glands secrete just the right amount of hormones; your heart beats and lungs breathe at the exact rate needed to supply oxygen to the rest of the body; your muscles contract to maintain balance and a steady temperature regardless of how you move or what the environmental temperature is; and, even your hair and fingernails grow at precise rates without your conscious awareness. There is a tremendous symphony of activity operating in harmony within your body without your conscious awareness. Trust this inner order as you become more aware of the dynamic stability and quiet intelligence within you.

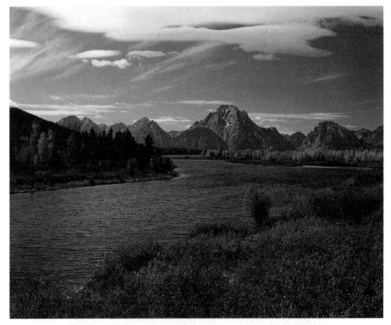

Used with permission from Microsoft

If centering seems foreign or difficult, recall a time when you were in a natural setting, such as the beach, a park, the mountains, or a still lake, where you felt a deep sense of peace, harmony, and relaxation. Affirm, "I AM that peace."

Soon you will notice your breathing becoming deeper and more relaxed, and muscular tension you had not even noticed will begin to melt. With practice, this state of inner quiet and harmonious integration, which is connected to the order and harmony within nature, will begin to feel like home, your own true self, which it is. When your mind wanders, call it back home.

Initially, it is easiest to practice centering for brief periods (one or two minutes) in a quiet, serene place. You may want to listen to uplifting music or soothing sounds from nature. Practicing with

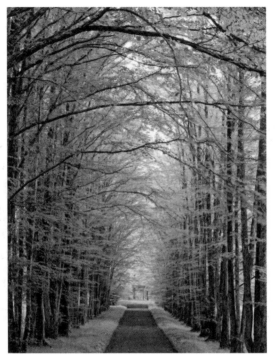

Used with permission from Microsoft

another person or a group of people also facilitates the centering process[11].

It may be helpful to use a portable biofeedback device, such as HeartMath's Personal Stress Reliever™, to confirm that you are in the "zone." Devices can be helpful, but they are not necessary. Regardless of the path you take, it is essential to develop confidence, based on your own experience, that you have an unshakable inner serenity that serves as a firm base from which to extend compassion.

---

11 An easy analogy is to think about singing. If you are trying to learn a new song, it is easier to sing along with a group that is singing that song, particularly if others in the group have sung it before.

Imagine the quiet depths of the sea; even if a storm moves the waves into a frothy pitch, the depths remain quiet.

For me, it has taken years of persistent practice in the face of numerous personal and professional challenges to achieve and maintain a sense of centeredness (and I can still "lose it" outside the context of healing work). I practice for 20 to 30 minutes every morning when it is quiet before I go to work, and I take several one-minute breaks throughout the day to re-focus on that inner serenity. I am a person with strong feelings, drive, and a long to-do list, so it is easy to get swept up in thoughts and emotions.

Before I enter a patient's room, I knock on the door, take a breath, reaffirm my intention to be helpful, and connect with the still, stable, orderly quiet within. As I open the door, I extend a sense of peace and goodwill, mentally offering to support the patient's goals for health and wellness. Washing hands before starting an examination or treatment also reminds me to wash away everything else and re-center myself so I can offer my very best to each patient[12].

Holding this strong center allows you to offer the strongest signal in the resonance of your relationships. As you hold this center, others around you will gradually become more peaceful themselves.

What Happens If You Lose Your Sense of Centeredness or the Conscious Connection with Your Inner Serenity?

Many healers are extremely sensitive to others, and if they lose their own centeredness, they begin to pick up the stress, anxiety, and

---

12 Please notice that I said "offer." We can offer goodwill and good advice, but it is the recipient's choice about taking either. Some patients reject every offer or idea with "yeah, but" excuses as to why it will not work for them. This rejection can be painful and lead to conflict and condemnation unless we remain centered in our inner serenity and unattached to the outcome.

KATHI J. KEMPER, M.D., M.P.H.

discomfort of those they are trying to help or their busy, distracted colleagues. They quickly feel out of sorts, tired, drained, irritable, or anxious themselves, and they have a hard time thinking clearly and extending compassion. Working without being centered is the fast track to burnout and ineffective care.

Other healers are better attuned to their own needs than those of others. Losing their center thrusts them back into self-interested thoughts (When will I do my grocery shopping, fold the laundry, pay bills?), distracting them from patients' needs. They may also begin to view patients as a means to achieve their own personal needs for understanding, support, or positive reinforcement, creating unfair, albeit unconscious, demands on patients.

A third type of healer is exquisitely aware of the environment and has a very flexible attention. While awareness and flexibility can be great strengths, if this kind of healer is not centered, it is very easy for the mind to wander to details of the room, the temperature, wall color, sounds, things happening outside the window, voices outside the door, or the emotions, attitudes, expressions, and activities of others who may be present or nearby. Distractions dissipate the energy and intention focused on the recipient, decreasing the effectiveness of the treatment. When this problem is severe, recipients may feel even more scattered and less supported than they did before the treatment began.

In short, failing to remain centered results in less-than-optimal outcomes for both healers and recipients.

Being centered means being keenly attuned to the serenity within. Practice centering in your inner, peaceful, quiet self. Spend time in nature. We will explore additional physical, mental, and spiritual strategies to strengthen centering in later chapters.

What Is Grounding?

Grounding

Electrically, grounding connects an electrical circuit to the earth. According to the National Electrical Code, a true earth ground consists of a conductive pipe or rod driven into the earth to a minimum depth of eight feet. For parental discipline, grounding means limiting activities to school, church, scouting, or home. In education, grounding refers to having a solid mastery of basic information in a field. Having a common ground means that people have a shared background or understanding. What do all these different definitions of grounding mean for healing?

For healers, the concept of grounding resonates with all these definitions. A healer is deeply connected or rooted to the intention to be helpful to others; whatever events transpire, this core intention is unshakable.

Being deeply rooted in a pure intention limits excursions into fantasy, excessive desires for praise, power or financial reward, lapses of laziness or impatience with the process, irritation with the recipient or other aspects of the situation, envy of other healers, and personal pride, arrogance, or self-aggrandizement. It helps the healer maintain a sense of humble curiosity and diligence. In order to be truly grounded, a healer must know herself (Chapter 1) and be willing to face and overcome both internal and external obstacles to achieving her deeply cherished goals to help others.

Being grounded means sharing an intention with the recipient for the highest and best outcome, whatever form that takes for a specific individual.

How Do You Get Grounded?

Physically, it's helpful to spend time sitting on the earth or a large rock; walking barefoot; leaning against a tree; strolling on the beach, allowing your feet to get wet; hiking in the hills; etc. Spending more time in nature and less time with electronic distractions can help reinforce your sense of being grounded.

Just as visualizing a harmonious, peaceful, restorative place in nature can help us center and settle into our quiet inner selves, visualizing can also help us become more grounded. Visualize yourself as an oak tree. Imagine your legs and feet extending deep into the earth. As they plunge into ever greater depths, tiny roots extend outward, holding onto the rich, rocky earth. Feel how firmly you are rooted in nurturing mother earth. No matter how windy, rainy, or stormy it is up in the branches, the roots remain still and strong. You are rooted in compassion, in the desire to help this person before you. You are part of a tremendous tradition reaching deep into human history. Whether the breezes of uncertainty blow, the raindrops of fantasy fall, or pride surges or storms, remember your roots and the nourishing wisdom of those who have humbly walked this path before you.

It may help to repeat this phrase to yourself as a meditation: "I am here only to be truly helpful."

Techniques and Effects

Whatever other techniques or tools you learn as a healer, they will serve you and those you seek to help best if you master the arts of centering and grounding. Simply being in the presence of someone who is centered and grounded is comforting, reassuring, and relaxing.

Regularly practicing centering and grounding can help healers feel better, too. Have doubts? That's okay. Let's review some of the research about the impact of different kinds of healing practices on healers and recipients.

CHAPTER 4

What Are the Types of Healing and What Are Their Effects on Recipients and Healers?

THIS CHAPTER DESCRIBES several common types of healing practices and the scientific evidence about their impact on the health of recipients and providers.

Types of Healing

Indigenous, traditional, and secular healing systems, as well as religions, have their own versions of healing. Indigenous healers around the world, sometimes called shamans, use a variety of tools to interact with the spirit world to access wisdom; eliminate noxious influences; and call on powerful allies and resources from the spirit world to help patients heal.

In addition to its better known practices of acupuncture and herbal medicine, Traditional Chinese Medicine includes the practice of external Qigong; a master healer transmits vital energy (Qi) to patients to help restore vitality, harmony, and balance. Such

KATHI J. KEMPER, M.D., M.P.H.

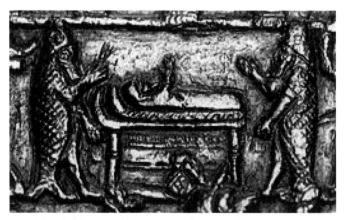

Lamashtu Healers, Assyria, Louvre, public access

practices actually predate acupuncture. Reiki and Johrei came from Japan. Ancient Ayurvedic hands-on healing practices from India have given rise to modern Polarity Therapy. Christianity refers to it as laying on of hands; Christian healers typically view themselves as channels of Divine healing power and may use music (hymns, chanting) and prayer to achieve a healing state (just as shamans use chanting and drumming).

After closely observing the Christian healers, Kathryn Kuhlman and Olga and Ambrose Worrall, and the lay healer, Colonel Oskar Estebany, Dora Kunz and Dolores Krieger, RN, developed a secular training for nurses called Therapeutic Touch. Additional healing practices have been developed by Americans Dr. W. Brugh Joy, Rosalyn Bruyere, Janet Mentgen (Healing Touch), Richard Gordon (Quantum Touch), Michael Bradford, Frank Kinslow, Barbara Brennan, Donna Eden, and others.

Although each practice has its own flavor and some of the personality of those who developed, taught, and wrote about it, these diverse healing practices share a common core of compassionate intention, dedication, and the healer's practice of putting self aside to focus on the recipient, extending goodwill and what is perceived as healing energy to support the dynamic drive toward order, harmony, and balance characteristic of health within the recipient. What impact do these different practices have on those who provide them?

Effects on the Healer

In 2010, our research team at Wake Forest Medical Center evaluated the impact of Healing Touch on nurses who began training. We found significant improvements in their stress, depression, anxiety, relaxation, well-being, and sleep[13]. Similar studies show decreased stress levels in nurses who learn and practice Reiki[14]. These findings confirm earlier studies showing that those who learn and practice Therapeutic Touch and other healing techniques tend to become more calm, relaxed, focused, and accepting over time[15]. Physiologically, studies have found significant changes in healers' heart rate patterns, EEG, skin temperature, and muscle tension[16]. Subjectively, they report feeling less stressed at work, a greater

13 Tang R., et al., "Improving the well-being of nursing leaders through healing touch training," *J Altern Complement Med.* 16, no.8 (2010): 837–41.

14 Cuneo C.L., "The effect of Reiki on work-related stress of the registered nurse," *J Holist Nurs.* 29, no. 1 (2011):33–43. Whelan KM, et al., "Reiki therapy: the benefits to a nurse/ Reiki practitioner," Holist Nurs Pract 17, no. 4 (2003): 209–17.

15 Lewis, D., "A survey of therapeutic touch practitioners," Nurs Stand 13, no. 30 (1999): 33–7.

16 Peper, E., et al., "The Two Endpoints of an EEG Continuum of Meditation Alpha/Theta and Fast Beta," Mind/Body Integration: Essential Readings in Biofeedback, E. Peper, S. Ancoli, and M. Quinn, Editors, (New York: Plenum, 1979), 141–148. Quinn JF, et al., "Psychoimmunologic effects of therapeutic touch on practitioners and recently bereaved recipients: a pilot study," *ANS Adv Nurs Sci* 15, no. 4 (1993): 13–26. Burleson KO, et al., "Energy healing training and heart rate variability," *J Altern Complement Med* 11, no. 3 (2005): 391–3.

KATHI J. KEMPER, M.D., M.P.H.

sense of self-esteem and spirituality, and more confidence in their ability to help others[17].

What Do Healers Feel in Their Hands When They Heal?

Healers engaged in healing work usually have a sense of energy, heat, fullness, or tingling in the hands. Sometimes as the hands are passed over a recipient, a healer gets a sense of heat, coolness, sharpness, waves, pulsing, tingling, pins and needles, pressure, bubbling, rhythmicity, fullness, or emptiness. At times the healer feels that the hands are being drawn to a place where there is difficulty. Sometimes healers will feel the recipient's pain or other symptoms in their own bodies. Those who are more keenly aware visually or more oriented to sound may not feel much in their hands, but rather notice subtle visual or auditory cues. Some have a sense of knowing or non-verbal awareness rather than a bodily sensation.

Does a Healer's Ability to Perceive Subtle Cues in the Recipient Affect Her Effectiveness?

Great question! Although sensing something in the recipient can be helpful for the healer to focus a particular treatment, it is not altogether clear that such sensations are necessary for a healing session to be beneficial. I have not found any research evaluating the relationship between what a healer perceives (in her hands or with other senses) and the impact of the healing session on the healer or the recipient (Wouldn't that be an interesting project?). It is possible that

---

17 Taylor B., et al., "The effects of Healing Touch on the coping ability, self esteem and general health of undergraduate nursing students," *Complement Ther Nurs Midwifery 7*, no. 1 (2001): 34–42. McElligott D., "A pilot feasibility study of the effects of touch therapy on nurses," *J N Y State Nurses Assoc.* 34, no. 1 (2003):16–24.

getting caught up in trying to perceive a particular sensation distracts from the central process. On the other hand, having a clearer sense of where and what kind of treatment is needed may help the healer make more informed, intelligent decisions and plans. Many healers report that their sensitivity and intuition improve over time naturally without being forced. Rather than focus on intensifying a particular perception, it is wise for healers to focus on centering, grounding, and extending peace, goodwill, and positive intentions, and releasing strong attachments to specific experiences or outcomes.

What Do Recipients Feel?

Just as there are differences in healers' perceptions, recipients may feel nothing at all or static electricity, heat, fullness, waves of energy, tingling, and easing of symptoms, such as pain, burning, nausea, or itch. Recipients may also sense sounds, music, or visual effects, such as colors, symbols, or light[18].

One of the best descriptions I've heard from a recipient came from a seven-year-old boy. He said that it felt like he was lying in a bathtub full of gelatin, and as my hands moved several inches over him, it felt like I was stroking the top of the gelatin and he could feel it jiggling on his skin.

Another vivid description came from a colleague who suffered from painful sinus congestion. As my fingers swept slowly past her cheeks and neck, she said it felt like there had been a large knot, and my fingers were gradually untangling the knot, smoothing the strands. Her face relaxed into a smile as the pain subsided and she freely took in several deep breaths through her previously congested nose.

---

18 Warber S., et al., "Biofield energy therapy: a qualitative study of the client's perspective," Alternative Therapies 15, no. 3 (2009) S159.

Do Recipients Ever Experience Negative Side Effects?

Yes, but rarely. Actually, side effects may help us appreciate the power of healing. Here are two confessions from my first ten years in practice that helped me understand the power of (poorly performed) healing practices to hurt as well as heal.

When I was a beginning student, I was given the opportunity to practice with a lovely older gentleman suffering from Parkinson's disease and a painful knee. He was sitting quite still as I began. Unaccustomed to the practice, I tried very hard to feel his energy field and then to send him energy. Within a few minutes, he began to tremble; within a few more minutes, the tremble turned into a pronounced tremor. The harder I tried, the more he shook. Fortunately, Dr. Susan Wager, a physician who was helping teach the class, saw what was happening and came over to help[19]. Although it looked to me like she was doing the exact same thing I was doing (sweeping hands slowly and lightly over his arms and legs), his tremor soon subsided. He didn't want to make me feel bad, but confessed that as I treated him, he felt more uncomfortable and ill at ease. Troubled at this failure, I asked Dr. Wager what I'd done "wrong." She told me, "You were just trying too hard. Remember to stay centered and relaxed during the process."

This is a terribly important lesson. *When we try too hard to feel something or forcefully send energy or try to achieve a very specific result, the recipient can feel worse.* Too much energy focused on the head can make a recipient feel spacey or disoriented. Too much energy over the throat can lead to sore throat or difficulty speaking. Trying too hard can backfire. Remain relaxed, curious, and unattached.

---

19 Dr. Wager is the author of *Doctor's Guide to Therapeutic Touch: Enhancing the Body's Energy to Promote Healing,* published by Perigree Books in 1996.

Here's another humbling example from my own experience. One day, I was in the Children's Hospital seeing a very sick baby who was attached to a ventilator (breathing machine) and numerous intravenous drips delivering life-saving medicine and nutrition. Her parents had requested Therapeutic Touch, and I was proud to offer it to her. The first couple of days were unremarkable. Then another healer asked to watch me treat her. Wanting to impress a colleague with my expertise, I tried very hard to "do it right." Within a minute, the baby's oxygen level fell, triggering an alarm. Startled, I pulled away. Her oxygen level rebounded. I took a deep breath and started again, reassuring myself that it was a coincidence and that I should just try harder. Again, her oxygen level fell as I treated her and improved when I stopped. A few days later, I went back to see her, without the distraction of trying to impress anyone else, and the session went off without a hitch. As her condition improved, and I continued to treat her, she relaxed more and more, falling asleep with higher oxygen levels within seconds of starting a session, even if she'd been crying vigorously when we started.

Of all the hundreds of patients I have treated over the years, these two impressed me the most. Why? *Because they showed that healing can have adverse effects when it is done improperly. If someone is trying too hard or trying to be impressive, she can cause unpleasant side effects. It is always important to monitor the patient and stop if things take a turn for the worse.* In medicine, we understand that powerful treatments can have serious side effects. Power is a two-edged sword. Seeing that healing work could have side effects helped me see its potential for helping, as well[20].

---

20 Dr. Shafica Karagulla also notes that "when healers are overenthusiastic and do not pay attention to their inner cues, they may pour too much energy into a patient with distressing and even harmful effects." *The Chakras and the Human Energy Fields,* (Quest Books, 1989), 180.

What Are the Most Common Benefits to Recipients?

Scientific studies show the primary benefit of healing is to promote relaxation, calm, ease, and comfort, while reducing stress, with greater improvements for patients treated by more experienced healers[21]. A conservative analysis of twenty-four studies (five for Healing Touch, sixteen of Therapeutic Touch, and three for Reiki) involving 1,153 participants showed an average improvement of about one point on a zero-to-ten scale of pain, with greater improvements noted among patients treated by more experienced healers[22]. There are no studies comparing one type of healing to another (e.g., spiritual healing vs. Reiki), so let's look at some of the main types of healing practiced in the United States today.

Effects of Therapeutic Touch (TT)

Therapeutic Touch was developed in 1972 by Dolores Krieger, R.N., Ph.D., and Dora Kunz. It has been described by its founders as a mode of "transpersonal healing" which involves "the knowledgeable use of innate therapeutic functions of the body to alleviate pain and combat illness." [23] This form of secular healing is most often provided by nurses, since one of the two founders (Krieger) was a professor of nursing at New York University. The practitioner consciously directs

---

21 Jackson, E., et al., "Does therapeutic touch help reduce pain and anxiety in patients with cancer?," Clin J Oncol Nurs 12, no. 1 (2008): 113–20. Kemper KJ, et al., "Treating children with therapeutic and healing touch," Pediatr Ann 33. no. 4 (2004): 248–52. MacIntyre B, et al., "The efficacy of healing touch in coronary artery bypass surgery recovery: a randomized clinical trial," Altern Ther Health Med 14, no. 4 (2008): 24–32.
22 So P.S., Jiang Y., Qin Y. Cochrane Database Syst Rev. 2008 Oct 8;(4):CD006535
23 Kunz D. and Krieger D., The Spiritual Dimension of Therapeutic Touch, (Bear and Company, 2004).

her vital energy to the recipient and assists the recipient in modulating his energy field to correct imbalances that manifest as illness.

Taught in over ninety countries in addition to the United States, TT is provided in over eighty medical centers in the United States by over 100,000 trained nurses. Because it was developed by an academic nurse, TT has undergone many research studies (initially by Krieger herself, and later by her graduate students, and then others). Dr. Krieger has noted that the sympathetic and parasympathetic nervous system (which balance the fight/flight response with rest/digest/tend/befriend activity) is the most sensitive body system to healing; the autonomic nervous system is followed by the lymphatic and circulatory systems, followed by muscles and connective tissues, joints, bones, and the central nervous system[24]. The numerous benefits of TT include relaxation, reduction of pain and stress, easing stress-related illnesses, and ramping up rate of recovery from injuries and surgery[25].

Therapeutic Touch has proven effective in reducing anxiety in patients with cancer and other serious illnesses[26]; it has also been useful in reducing pain and anxiety in children[27]; TT can also improve

---

24 Krieger, D., "Dolores Krieger, RN, PhD healing with therapeutic touch," Interview by Bonnie Horrigan, *Altern Ther Health Med* 4, no 1.(1998):86–92.
25 Coakley AB, et al., "The effect of therapeutic touch on postoperative patients," *J Holist Nurs* 28, no. 3 (2010): 193–200.
26 Jackson, E., et al., "Does therapeutic touch help reduce pain and anxiety in patients with cancer?,: *Clin J Oncol Nurs* 12, no. 1 (2008): 113–20. Giasson, M, et al., "Effect of therapeutic touch on the well-being of persons with terminal cancer," *J Holist Nurs* 16, no. 3 (1998): 383–98. Aghabati, NE, et al., "The Effect of Therapeutic Touch on Pain and Fatigue of Cancer Patients Undergoing Chemotherapy," *Evid Based Complement Alternat Med*, (2008). Aghabati, NE, et al., "The Effect of Therapeutic Touch on Pain and Fatigue of Cancer Patients Undergoing Chemotherapy, *Evid Based Complement Alternat Med*, (2008).
27 Kemper K.J., et al., "Treating children with therapeutic and healing touch," *Pediatr Ann* 33, no. 4 (2004): 248–52.

mood and anxiety in adults[28] ; and it can reduce restlessness among Alzheimer's patients[29] and patients in intensive care units[30]. It can also ease the pain of arthritis[31].

Most studies on healing work have been conducted in healthy people or medical settings, but this approach can be helpful with mental and emotional health, too. A study from the United Kingdom showed significant improvements in stress, anxiety, depression, relaxation, and ability to cope among 147 clients who had self-identified mental health problems[32]. It has also been used successfully to soothe symptoms in patients undergoing treatment for addictions[33].

---

28 Lafreniere K.D., et al., "Effects of therapeutic touch on biochemical and mood indicators in women," *J Altern Complement Med* 5, no. 4 (1999): 367–70. Larden, C.N., et al., "Efficacy of therapeutic touch in treating pregnant inpatients who have a chemical dependency," *J Holist Nurs* 22, no. 4 (2004): 320–32. Simington JA, et al., "Effects of therapeutic touch on anxiety in the institutionalized elderly," *Clin Nurs Res* 2, no. 4 (1993): 438–50. Gagne D, et al., "The effects of therapeutic touch and relaxation therapy in reducing anxiety," *Arch Psychiatr Nurs* 8, no. 3 (1994): 184–9. Robinson J, et al., "Therapeutic touch for anxiety disorders," *Cochrane Database Syst Rev,* 2007(3): CD006240.
29 Woods D.L., et al., "The effect of therapeutic touch on agitated behavior and cortisol in persons with Alzheimer's disease," *Biol Res Nurs* 4, no. 2 (2002):104–14. Woods DL, et al., "The effect of therapeutic touch on behavioral symptoms and cortisol in persons with dementia," *Forsch Komplementmed* 16, no. 3 (2009): 181–9.
30 Cox C., et al., "Experiences of administering and receiving therapeutic touch in intensive care," *Complement Ther Nurs Midwifery* 4, no. 5 (1998): 128–32.
31 Gordon A., et al., "The effects of therapeutic touch on patients with osteoarthritis of the knee," *J Fam Pract* 47, no. 4 (1998): 271–7. Peck S.D., "The efficacy of therapeutic touch for improving functional ability in elders with degenerative arthritis.,"*Nurs Sci Q* 11, no. 3 (1998): 123–32.
32 Weze, C., et al., "Healing by Gentle Touch Ameliorates Stress and Other Symptoms in People Suffering with Mental Health Disorders or Psychological Stress," *Evid Based Complement Alternat Med* 4, no. 1 (2007): 115–123.
33 Hagemaster J., "Use of therapeutic touch in treatment of drug addictions," *Holist Nurs Pract* 14, no. 3 (2000): 14–20. Larden C.N., et al., "Efficacy of therapeutic touch in treating pregnant inpatients who have a chemical dependency," *J Holist Nurs* 22, no. 4 (2004): 320–32.

Effects of Healing Touch (HT)

Healing Touch was developed in the 1990s by a nurse, Janet Mentgen, RN, BSN, as an outgrowth of other techniques, such as TT and practices promulgated by American healers, Dr. Brugh Joy, Barbara Brennan, and Rosalyn Bruyere. Healing Touch includes several non-invasive techniques to clear and balance the human energy fields to restore, energize, and rebalance human energy fields. Over 150,000 people worldwide have studied HT, and there are over 3,000 certified HT practitioners who have completed the five levels of training.

Healing Touch is most commonly used to help relieve pain and fatigue, distressed breathing, fear and anxiety, and spiritual distress; to promote overall health and well-being and enhance wound healing; and assist in recovering from symptoms related to exposure to toxins and chemotherapy.

As with TT, studies on HT suggest it can reduce pain for several conditions, including post-surgical pain in children[34], severe recurrent headaches[35], veterans with chronic pain[36], and cancer patients[37].

Anxiety and stress also respond well to HT. For example, patients undergoing heart surgery had less anxiety and shorter hospital stays when they received HT[38]. A single HT treatment can lower both anxiety and physiologic measures of stress (heart rate, blood

---

34 Zimmer M.M., "Effect of healing touch on children's pain and comfort in the postoperative period," Explore (NY) 5, (2009): 157.

35 Sutherland E.G., et al., "An HMO-based prospective pilot study of energy medicine for chronic headaches: whole-person outcomes point to the need for new instrumentation," J Altern Complement Med 15, no. 8 (2009): 819–26.

36 Wardell D.W., et al., "Study descriptions of healing touch with veterans experiencing chronic neuropathic pain from spinal cord injury," Explore (NY) 4, no. 3 (2008): 187–95.

37 Post-White J., et al., "Therapeutic massage and healing touch improve symptoms in cancer," Integr Cancer Ther 2, no. 4 (2003): 332–44. Cook C.A., et al., "Healing touch and quality of life in women receiving radiation treatment for cancer: a randomized controlled trial," Altern Ther Health Med 10, no. 3 (2004): 34–41.

38 MacIntyre B., et al., Altern Ther Health Med 14, no. 4 (2008): 24–32.

pressure, skin conductance, and skin temperature)[39]. Stress is a well-known risk factor for immune dysfunction and mood problems. In a 2010 study, HT treatments were superior to usual care or relaxation training for women with cervical cancer who were undergoing chemotherapy and radiation in terms of preserving immune function and preventing depression[40].

Treatments with HT have also improved the quality of life during treatment for cancer[41]. Our study at Wake Forest showed that HT treatments helped pediatric oncology patients reduce anxiety levels[42]. Another Wake Forest study showed decreased nausea and improved fatigue among adult oncology patients who received HT[43].

Experience counts. Improvements are generally, though not always, greater with treatments from experienced than novice practitioners[44].

Benefits of Reiki and Johrei

As with TT, the autonomic (sympathetic and parasympathetic) nervous system appears to be among the most sensitive of the body's

---

39 Maville J.A., et al., "Effect of Healing Touch on stress perception and biological correlates," *Holist Nurs Pract* 22, no. 2 (2008):103–10.

40 Lutgendorf S.K., et al., "Preservation of immune function in cervical cancer patients during chemoradiation using a novel integrative approach," Brain Behav Immun 24, no. 8 (2010) :1231–40.

41 Cook C.A., et al., "Healing touch and quality of life in women receiving radiation treatment for cancer: a randomized controlled trial," *Altern Ther Health Med* 10, no. 3 (2004):34–41.

42 Kemper K.J., et al., "Impact of healing touch on pediatric oncology outpatients: pilot study," *J Soc Integr Oncol*, 7, no. 1 (2009):12–8.

43 Danhauer S., et al., "Healing Touch as a Supportive Intervention for Adult Acute Leukemia Patients: A Pilot Investigation of Effects on Distress and Symptoms," *JSIO* 6, no. 3 (2008): 89–97.

44 Wilkinson D.S., et al., "The clinical effectiveness of healing touch," *J Altern Complement Med* 8, no. 1 (2002):33–47.

systems in response to Reiki[45]. That is, Reiki promotes parasympathetic (rest and digest) activity and decreases sympathetic (fight or flight) activity.

Reiki reduces anxiety and stress hormones, even in healthy people who are not particularly stressed, as well as in patients undergoing surgery and procedures (who also experience less pain and use fewer pain medications when they receive Reiki)[46]. For example, Reiki treatment improved physiologic measures of anxiety among adults who underwent screening colonoscopy[47]. It can also reduce stress in children[48].

Similarly, among older adults with pain, anxiety, or depression, Reiki treatment improved relaxation, comfort, and mood, as well as anxiety[49]. As with TT and HT, Reiki treatments can also help reduce pain and fatigue, improving the quality of life of patients with cancer[50]. Weekly Reiki treatments significantly improved mental functioning and memory over four weeks in a small study of older adults[51].

---

45 Friedman, R.S., et al., "Effects of Reiki on autonomic activity early after acute coronary syndrome," *J Am Coll Cardiol* 56, no. 12 (2010): 995–6. Mackay N.S., et al., "Autonomic nervous system changes during Reiki treatment: a preliminary study," *J Altern Complement Med* 10, no. 6 (2004): 1077–81.

46 Vitale A.T., et al., "The effect of Reiki on pain and anxiety in women with abdominal hysterectomies: a quasi-experimental pilot study," *Holist Nurs Pract* 20, no. 6 (2006): 263–72. Friedman R.S., et al., "Effects of Reiki on autonomic activity early after acute coronary syndrome," *J Am Coll Cardiol* 56, no. 12 (2010): 995–6. Thrane S., Cohen S.M., "Effect of Reiki Therapy on Pain and Anxiety in Adults: An In-Depth Literature Review of Randomized Trials with Effect Size Calculations," *Pain Manag Nurs* (2014): S1524–9042.

47 Hulse R.S., et al., "Endoscopic procedure with a modified Reiki intervention: a pilot study," *Gastroenterol Nurs* 33, no. 1 (2010): 20–6.

48 Bukowski E.L., Berardi D., "Reiki brief report: using reiki to reduce stress levels in a nine-year-old child," *Explore* (NY) 10, no. 4 (2014):253–5.

49 Richeson N.E., et al., "Effects of Reiki on anxiety, depression, pain, and physiological factors in community-dwelling older adults," *Res Gerontol Nurs* 3, no. 3 (2010):187–99.

50 Olson K.J., et al., "A phase II trial of Reiki for the management of pain in advanced cancer patients," *J Pain Symptom* Manage 25, no. 5 (2003): 990–7.

51 Crawford S.E., et al., "Using Reiki to decrease memory and behavior problems in mild cognitive impairment and mild Alzheimer's disease," *J Altern Complement Med* 12, no. 9 (2006): 911–3.

Another Japanese healing practice is *Johrei*. Although less research has been done on this practice than with Reiki, similar benefits have been noted for the practitioner and the recipient: more emotional well-being and decreased pain and stress[52]. Johrei treatments also helped substance abusers in twelve-step programs experience less distress and better mood than other patients who did not receive Johrei[53].

However, not all studies on Reiki or Johrei have shown positive effects[54]. In a small study of children undergoing dental procedures, true Reiki treatment failed to reduce pain any more than sham Reiki treatment[55]. Likewise, in a study of 189 people receiving outpatient chemotherapy, having a supportive nurse present was just as effective as a Reiki treatment in raising levels of comfort and well-being[56]. And a set of eight experiments in which Johrei healers attempted to influence the growth of cancer cells in a laboratory showed no observable effects[57].

Much more research is needed to better understand how these therapies work, in what situations, and for what conditions they are most helpful.

---

52 Laidlaw T.M., et al., The influence of 10 min of the Johrei healing method on laboratory stress," *Complement Ther Med* 14, no. 2 (2006): 127–32. Reece K., et al., "Positive well-being changes associated with giving and receiving Johrei healing," *J Altern Complement Med* 11, no. 3 (2005): 455–7.
53 Brooks A.J., et al., "The effect of Johrei healing on substance abuse recovery: a pilot study," *J Altern Complement Med* 12, no. 7 (2006): 625–31.
54 Hall Z., et al., "Radiation response of cultured human cells is unaffected by Johrei," *Evid Based Complement Alternat Med* 4, no. 2 (2007):191–4.
55 Kundu A., et al., "Reiki therapy for postoperative oral pain in pediatric patients: pilot data from a double-blind, randomized clinical trial," *Complement Ther Clin Pract* 20, no. 1 (2014):21–5.
56 Catlin A., Taylor-Ford R.L., "Investigation of standard care versus sham Reiki placebo versus actual Reiki therapy to enhance comfort and well-being in a chemotherapy infusion center," *Oncol Nurs Forum* 38, no. 3 (2011):E212–20.
57 Taft R., et al., "Time-lapse analysis of potential cellular responsiveness to Johrei, a Japanese healing technique," *BMC Complement Altern Med*, (2005), 5:2.

Studies on Qigong

The ancient Chinese practice of Qigong has developed into numerous schools and techniques[58]. The two main types of practice are internal Qigong, which is a moving meditation similar to tai chi, and external or medical Qigong, in which a master practitioner emits Qi toward a patient to promote healing. Although Qigong is an ancient practice, it was suppressed during the cultural revolution of the 1960s, and modern scientific research about it did not get underway until the later 1970s and 1980s. Since then, hundreds of studies have documented the benefits of external Qigong for treating patients with a variety of painful conditions, only a few of which have been translated into English[59].

Much of the early research tried to understand the energy emitted by Qigong healers—patterns of low-frequency modulated infrared radiation, electromagnetic radiation, infrasonic radiation, etc., emitted from master healer's hands. Studies support each of these mechanisms, but a unifying theory remains elusive.

One of the challenges in research on external Qigong is that unlike other traditions, in which healers draw upon universal healing energy, Qigong masters typically draw upon their own personal qi energy to heal. This means that when an experiment is repeated

---

58 Beijing alone has nearly two dozen schools of Qigong, including New Qigong, Wild Goose Qigong, Flying Crane Qigong, Six-Character Qigong, Standing Qigong, and self-adjustment Qigong. Millions of Chinese people practice Qigong outdoors in parks daily.
59 Chen K.W., et al., "An analytic review of studies on measuring effects of external QI in China," Altern Ther Health Med 10, no. 4 (2004): 38–50. Chen K.W., et al., "A pilot study of external qigong therapy for patients with fibromyalgia," J Altern Complement Med 12, no. 9 (2006): 851–6. Lee M.S., et al., "External Qi therapy to treat symptoms of Agent Orange Sequelae in Korean combat veterans of the Vietnam War," Am J Chin Med 32, no. 3 (2004): 461–6. Lee M.S., et al., "Effects of Qi-therapy on blood pressure, pain and psychological symptoms in the elderly: a randomized controlled pilot trial," Complement Ther Med 11, no. 3 (2003): 159–64.

several times in one day, the healer tires, and effects diminish[60]. This makes it difficult to achieve the large sample sizes and consistent outcomes that characterize compelling biomedical research.

Despite this limitation, studies show that Qigong healers can improve pain and anxiety for patients with severe, chronic pain[61], including fibromyalgia[62], premenstrual pain[63], and osteoarthritis, though there is variability in the effectiveness of different Qigong healers, as with other types of therapists[64].

Also similar to other types of healing, Qigong appears to affect not just symptoms, but the underlying physiology of the autonomic nervous system, slowing the heart rate and increasing heart rate variability, suggesting increased vagal tone[65].

Polarity Therapy (PT)

Polarity Therapy was developed in the 1940s and '50s by American chiropractor and osteopath, Randolph Stone. Like Therapeutic and Healing Touch, Reiki and Johrei, and Qigong, PT is based on a belief

---

60 Yount G., et al., "In vitro test of external Qigong," BMC Complement Altern Med (2004), Mar 15; 4:5.

61 Lee M.S., et al., "External qigong for pain conditions: a systematic review of randomized clinical trials," J Pain 8, no. 11 (2007): 827–31. Wu W.H., et al., "Effects of qigong on late-stage complex regional pain syndrome," Altern Ther Health Med, 1999; 5(1): 45–54

62 Chen KW, et al., A pilot study of external qigong therapy for patients with fibromyalgia. J Altern Complement Med 12, no. 9 (2006): 851–6.

63 Jang H.S., et al., "Effects of qi therapy (external qigong) on premenstrual syndrome: a randomized placebo-controlled study," J Altern Complement Med 10, no. 3 (2004): 456–62.

64 Chen K.W., et al., "Effects of external qigong therapy on osteoarthritis of the knee. A randomized controlled trial," Clin Rheumatol 27, no. 12 (2008): 1497–505. Vincent A. et al., "External qigong for chronic pain," Am J Chin Med 38, no. 4 (2010): 695–703.

65 Lee M.S., et al., "Effects of Qi-therapy (external Qigong) on cardiac autonomic tone: a randomized placebo controlled study," Int J Neurosci 115, no.9 (2005):1345–50.

in an energy field that permeates the human body that can be influenced to improve health.

A 1999 Ohio study examined whether gamma radiation might be a mechanism for the observed benefits of Polarity Therapy. Researchers found decreased gamma radiation in subjects' electromagnetic fields when they were exposed to Polarity Therapy compared with simple rest and sham conditions[66]. This does not necessarily prove that gamma radiation plays a major role in the mechanism, but it is intriguing and points out the need for additional research on mechanisms of effects. What about clinical effects?

In a study of breast cancer patients undergoing radiation therapy and experiencing fatigue, weekly Polarity Therapy (PT) treatments were associated with a significant improvement in fatigue and quality of life compared with mock treatments or no PT[67]. These benefits were confirmed in a later study in which PT was as effective as massage and both were more helpful than treatment as usual (without these complementary therapies) for patients receiving radiation therapy[68].

Similarly, Polarity Therapy proved more effective than a comparison intervention in improving stress, pain, vitality, and general health among caregivers of dementia patients[69].

---

66 Benford M.S., et al., "Gamma radiation fluctuations during alternative healing therapy," *Altern Ther Health Med* 5, no. 4 (1999): 51–6.
67 Roscoe J.A., et al., "Treatment of radiotherapy-induced fatigue through a nonpharmacological approach," *Integr Cancer Ther* 4, no. 1 (2005): 8–13.
68 Mustian K.M., et al., "Polarity Therapy for cancer-related fatigue in patients with breast cancer receiving radiation therapy: a randomized controlled pilot study," *Integr Cancer Ther* 10, no. 1 (2011): 27–37.
69 Korn L., et al., "A randomized trial of a CAM therapy for stress reduction in American Indian and Alaskan Native family caregivers," *Gerontologist* 49, no. 3 (2009): 368–77.

Spiritual Healing, Gentle Touch with Intention, and Healing Prayer

There is a huge body of human experience with many varieties of spiritual healing, laying on of hands, gentle touch[70], and healing prayer. Results of the scientific studies on these practices have been somewhat mixed, but are generally similar to the results from TT, HT, Reiki, Johrei, and Qigong in terms of improvements in pain, anxiety, and overall well-being[71].

Studies on the effects of intercessory prayer or distant prayer healing have had mixed results[72].

Shamanic or Indigenous Healing Practices

Shamanic healing has become the term used for indigenous healing practices and rituals around the world that draw on a sense of sacred connection with the natural world. Shamans enter an altered state of consciousness to communicate with the spirits and unseen energies,

---

70 Weze, C., et al., "Evaluation of healing by gentle touch in 35 clients with cancer," Eur J Oncol Nurs 8, no. 1 (2004): 40–9.

71 Jonas W.B. and Crawford CC.., "Science and spiritual healing: a critical review of spiritual healing, "energy" medicine, and intentionality," Altern Ther Health Med 9, no. 2 (2003): 56–61. Levin J., et al., "Bioenergy healing: a theoretical model and case series," Explore (NY) 4, no. 3 (2008): 201–9.

72 Krucoff M.W., et al., "Music, imagery, touch, and prayer as adjuncts to interventional cardiac care: the Monitoring and Actualization of Noetic Trainings (MANTRA) II randomized study," Lancet 366, no. 9481 (2005): 211–7. Benson H., et al., "Study of the Therapeutic Effects of Intercessory Prayer (STEP) in cardiac bypass patients: a multicenter randomized trial of uncertainty and certainty of receiving intercessory prayer," Am Heart J 151, no. 4 (2006):934–42. Moga M.M., et al., "Distant healing of small-sized tumors," J Altern Complement Med 14, no. 5 (2008): 453. Radin D., et al., "Compassionate intention as a therapeutic intervention by partners of cancer patients: effects of distant intention on the patients' autonomic nervous system," Explore (NY) 4, no. 4 (2008): 235–43. Tsubono K.P., et al., "The effects of distant healing performed by a spiritual healer on chronic pain: a randomized controlled trial," Altern Ther Health Med 15, no. 3 (2009): 30–4. Roberts L., et al., "Intercessory prayer for the alleviation of ill health," Cochrane Database Syst Rev, 2009(2): CD000368.

sometimes using drumming or chanting, and sometimes with the assistance of potent herbs. Shamans may communicate with plants to identify those useful for healing, help dispel negative energies, or call on powerful spiritual allies to achieve healing purposes.

Although these concepts might appear primitive and foreign to modern Westerners, researchers at Kaiser Permanente in Portland, Oregon, undertook a study of the effects of shamanic healing for patients with a modern malady—temporomandibular joint disease (TMJ). In the first study, of twenty-three women diagnosed with TMJ, a series of five shamanic healing sessions led to a dramatic improvement in pain, such that by the end of the study, only four of the women still met criteria for diagnosis[73]. In a follow-up study, researchers found that although the physical improvements were impressive, the women who received shamanic healing reported even greater improvements in self-awareness, capacity for coping, the quality of their interpersonal relationships, and capacity for self-care[74]; these benefits persisted over nine months of follow-up. Altogether, these studies point to a transformational, holistic healing experience that encompassed far more than physical health.

Are Benefits Just the Placebo Effect?

Although skeptics might claim that the benefits are only due to a placebo effect, this opinion is refuted by findings from cell culture studies[75]. As far as we know, cells in test tubes and petri dishes are

---

73 Vuckovic N.H., et al., "Feasibility and short-term outcomes of a shamanic treatment for temporomandibular joint disorders," *Altern Ther Health Med* 13, no. 6 (2007):18–29.
74 Vuckovic N., et al., "Journey into healing: the transformative experience of shamanic healing on women with temporomandibular joint disorders," *Explore (NY)* 6, no. 6 (2010):371–9.
75 Savieto R.M., et al., "Therapeutic touch for the healing of skin injuries in guinea pigs," *Rev Bras Enferm* 57, no. 3 (2004): 340–3.

not susceptible to placebo effects. However, studies at the University of Connecticut have shown that Therapeutic Touch treatments have a dramatic impact on the growth and metabolism of bone, connective tissue, and tendon cells growing in laboratory cultures. In human bone cells, Therapeutic Touch increased DNA synthesis, differentiation, and mineralization, and decreased differentiation and mineralization in a human osteosarcoma (cancer)-derived cell lines[76]. A study on premature infants (who are also unlikely to be affected by placebos), showed improved balance in the autonomic nervous system governing heart rate and breathing among those who received TT[77].

Similarly, the benefits of Johrei appear to be more than just placebo effects. A study in mice confirmed significant benefits on sleep under stressful conditions in those who received Johrei compared with those who did not[78]. Likewise, Johrei impacted the growth of cancer cells in test tubes[79]. This is not to claim that Johrei or Reiki are cures for cancer, but that they have effects in test tube studies that cannot be explained on the basis of psychological or placebo mechanisms.

Furthermore, Qigong master healers have demonstrated significant effects on biophysical systems, such as liquid crystal arrays, cell membranes, water, saline, atomic nuclear radioactive decay

---

76 Gronowicz G.A., et al., "Therapeutic touch stimulates the proliferation of human cells in culture," J Altern Complement Med 14, no. 3 (2008): 233–9. Jhaveri A., et al., "Therapeutic touch affects DNA synthesis and mineralization of human osteoblasts in culture," J Orthop Res 26, no. 11 (2008):1541–6.

77 Whitley J.A., et al., "A double-blind randomized controlled pilot trial examining the safety and efficacy of therapeutic touch in premature infants," Adv Neonatal Care 8, no. 6 (2008): 315–33.

78 Buzzetti R.A., et al., "Effect of Johrei therapy on sleep in a murine model," Explore (NY) 9, no. 2 (2013): 100–5.

79 Abe K., et al., "Effect of a Japanese energy healing method known as Johrei on viability and proliferation of cultured cancer cells in vitro," J Altern Complement Med 18, no. 3 (2012): 221–8.

rates, RNA, DNA, collagen, hemoglobin, and albumin[80]. Preliminary studies in tissue cultures and in mice have shown decreases in tumors for mice treated by Qigong masters[81].

In summary, there are many different kinds of healing practices from the world's many different cultures. Despite their obvious differences, these practices have similar benefits for healers and recipients: increased relaxation and well-being, and decreased stress and pain. Sounds good, right? What are the basic requirements for getting started and how do you prepare to be a healer? That's what Part 2 is all about.

---

80 Chen K.W., "An analytic review of studies on measuring effects of external QI in China," *Altern Ther Health Med* 10, no. 4 (2004): 38–50. Lu Zuyin, *Scientific QiGong Exploration*, (Amber Leaf Press, 1997).

81 Yan X., et al., "External Qi of Yan Xin Qigong Induces apoptosis and inhibits migration and invasion of estrogen-independent breast cancer cells through suppression of Akt/NF-kB signaling," *Cell Physiol Biochem* 25, no 23 (2010): 263–70. Yan X,, et al., "External Qi of Yan Xin Qigong induces G2/M arrest and apoptosis of androgen-independent prostate cancer cells by inhibiting Akt and NF-kappa B pathways," *Mol Cell Biochem* 310, no. 12 (2008):227–34.

PART 2

Preparation for Healing

CHAPTER 5

Basic Requirements and Physical Preparation

YOU PROBABLY ALREADY HAVE the basic requirements for healing. Let's just review those and some ways we can prepare our bodies to be better vehicles for healing work. You don't need to be perfect, but it is helpful to have high ideals for this sacred work. The basic requirements for practicing healing are simple:

- Compassion: the desire to relieve another's suffering
- Loving-kindness: the desire for another to experience well-being
- Good health: physical vitality and resilience; mental and emotional cheerfulness, calmness, and peacefulness; spiritually, having a sense of meaning, purpose, and connection to something greater than one's conscious self (e.g., purpose, ethics, community, God, nature)
- Self-awareness, self-discipline, dedication, and sincerity: willingness to look over your own shoulder to become master of yourself, your thoughts, and emotions; ability to overcome fear, anger, resentment, pride, and jealousy; and willingness to learn from others and from experience
- Mental focus: the ability to control attention and maintain

multiple types of awareness simultaneously (e.g., the ability to remain centered while attending to another's changing needs)

- Stability, equanimity, and resilience in the face of chaos, confusion, change, and challenge
- Courage and willingness to confront barriers within self to becoming more effective
- Curiosity, flexibility, and openness to learning about being a participant in the healing process rather than relying on dogma
- Honesty and tact: offering hope and good cheer without setting up unrealistic expectations
- Non-judgmental acceptance of self, others, and the process: being willing to accept and learn from whatever arises, including the unexpected
- Humility and respect. Healers hold a collaborative, empowering attitude, working in a respectful partnership with the person seeking help, not attempting to dominate or control the person or the outcome. Healers ask permission. They avoid making assumptions
- Confidence and trust in the strength of one's quiet inner self, the source of intuition, common sense, and practicality
- Detachment: while maintaining compassion, the healer remains detached from the specific results and does not claim credit for the results, knowing that ultimately, healing is up to the person seeking help, nature, and the environment in which the person lives.

Healers do not need to be perfect, but just as athletes aim for rigorous training and optimal conditions to achieve peak performance, healers need to be aware of and cultivate the optimal training and conditions for healing.

Dolores Krieger warned against the "four dragons" that healers must mentally guard against: wishful thinking, impulse, fantasy, and exaggeration[82]. What do we need to guard against, and to what should we pay attention?

Guard Against	Pay Attention to Real Cues
Wishful thinking	Pay attention to physical cues and what the recipient says and does. Pay attention to the surroundings. Note if the sun is shining or there is an air vent that may be contributing to sensations of warmth or coolness. Watch the recipient's breathing rate, facial expressions, skin color, muscle tone, sweating, posture, restlessness, or calmness.
Impulsivity	Do an assessment and make a plan before starting a treatment.
Fantasy	Seek feedback from the recipient and other caregivers; compare your observations with others and with monitors, laboratory tests, and imaging studies when available.
Exaggerated self-importance; trying to impress others with your abilities	Credit the recipient, nature, your teachers and training; avoid taking personal credit for positive outcomes.
Exaggerated self-doubt	Maintain confidence in your intuition, training, experience, and the innate healing ability present in each person.
Over-Treatment/trying too hard	Watch for signs of excess treatment, such as restlessness. If the recipient becomes irritable, anxious, hostile, or reports increasing pain, fullness, itchiness, nausea, light-headedness, or spaciness, stop treatment.
Laziness	Maintain dedication and focus on healing rather than being distracted by the general busyness of the world. Ask yourself what you can do to help, rather than wait for others to initiate assistance.

---

82 Krieger D., *Therapeutic Touch as Transpersonal Healing*, (New York: Lantern/Book-Light, 2002).

Embracing the Paradox

Healers embrace the mystery and the fundamental paradoxes of healing. That is, healers:

- Do not heal (recipients do)
- Have clear intention to be helpful (yet remain unattached to results)
- Remain centered on the internal timeless equilibrium of universal peace and wholeness (yet are aware of the recipient's changing needs and the impact of the treatment on the recipient)
- Engage in effortless effort (avoid excessive effort, remain relaxed and accepting while working for something better)

Physical Preparation

One of the key essentials of being an effective healer is being healthy and relaxed, filled with vitality and resilience. Do not attempt to offer healing to someone else when you feel debilitated, fatigued, hungry, in pain, overwhelmed, depressed, stressed, anxious, afraid, envious, angry, or scattered. It is important for healers to take good care of their own health.

Is a Special Diet Necessary?

Not necessarily, but do make sure you get *good nutrition*. Some healers feel that it is important to avoid using stimulants or sedatives themselves (avoiding coffee, tobacco, alcohol, and mood-altering drugs). Others feel it is essential to adhere to a vegetarian or vegan diet to embody the principle of harmlessness to all sentient beings.

There are no studies comparing the effectiveness of healers who partake of different foods. However, it makes sense that if you violate your own sense of a right and proper diet, your guilt may impair your ability to be effective. If you try to heal when hungry or just after a large meal, you may be distracted by your own tummy rumbling or sense of satiated lethargy.

Do I Have to Become an Athlete?

No, but regular exercise and optimal amounts of sleep also promote the sense of vitality, strength, stamina, balance, and flexibility that are helpful for a healer to function at his best. Consider studying yoga, tai chi, or Qigong to build mindful awareness of your body. Regular exercises of this nature promote greater awareness of oneself and awareness of the prana or qi—Eastern concepts of life force or life energy. Regular exercise in natural settings builds a sense of connection to natural sources of strength and healing.

Personally, I practice yoga in addition to regular aerobic exercise and strength training to improve my stamina, strength, and balance. Also, because I spend a lot of time "in my head," practicing yoga helps me re-connect with my physical body. Practicing Tai Chi helps me maintain an awareness of the benefits of coordinating movement with slow, deep breathing, while promoting balance and flexibility.

Does this mean you need to train for a marathon or become a yogi? No, but common sense suggests that trying to help someone else when you feel lethargic and fatigued is unlikely to yield optimal results.

Do I Have to Avoid Ever Having Strong Emotions?

No, just like hunger, thirst, and fatigue, emotions are part of the human experience. However, most healers also find it helpful to regularly engage in practices that promote optimal mental and emotional self-regulation and stress management to promote mental and emotional resilience in the face of the suffering encountered in healing practice. Consider practicing mindful eating, gazing, walking, and breathing to promote mindful self-awareness, acceptance, and open-hearted, friendly curiosity throughout your daily activities.

Nurturing positive, supportive, restorative relationships also helps create a mental and emotional reserve to buffer against stress and supply solid, grounded energy.

Progressive Muscle Relaxation (PMR)

Progressive muscle relaxation is one of the easiest, most well-known ways to promote relaxation. It does not require any special equipment. Simply tighten a set of muscles, hold, and release; then progress to the next set of muscles. The only decision you need to make is whether to start with the muscles of the scalp and work your way down, or start with the muscles in your feet and work your way up. I generally start with my feet.

1. Notice the sensations in your feet and toes.
2. Tighten the muscles. Tight. Tight. Tight. Hold it for five to ten seconds. Breathe.
3. Now relax the muscles off the feet and toes. Ahh.
4. Next tighten the ankles. Tight. Tight. Tight. Hold it. Breathe.
5. Now relax the muscles of the ankles. Breathe.
6. And so forth, up the legs, to the hips, buttocks, lower back, middle and upper back, belly, chest, neck, hands, arms, shoulders, neck, face and jaw, forehead, and scalp.
7. When you've finished, mentally scan your body, noting any

areas of remaining tension.

8. Go ahead and tighten them one by one again, breathing and releasing until everything is nice and relaxed. For particularly tense areas, you may repeat the process three to four times. It gets easier the more you practice.

9. The whole process generally takes ten to twenty minutes.

10. Want to listen to a guided recording of the progressive muscle relaxation process for free? Go to the Ohio State University Center for Integrative Health and Wellness web site: http://go.osu.edu/guidedimagerypractices. And scroll down to Patrice Rancour's recording of Progressive Muscle Relaxation. You can download the MP3 file to your smart device to listen any time you like.

    Dartmouth College also has free recordings on their website: http://www.dartmouth.edu/~healthed/relax/down loads.html

    So does the McKinley Health Center at the University of Illinois: http://www.mckinley.illinois.edu/units/health_ed/ elax_relaxation_exercises.htm

    You can also find plenty of YouTube recordings if you prefer video.

    If you want to learn from a teacher in person, check with a certified yoga teacher or licensed counselor or psychologist in your area.

Autogenic Training: Fostering Deep Relaxation

Autogenic training was developed by a German psychiatrist in the 1930s as a brief (fifteen-minute) practice to enhance relaxation. Norman Shealy, M.D., Ph.D., one of the founders of the American Holistic Medical Association, taught me this technique when I was in medical school. I still use it. Autogenic training consists of the repetition of a series of six simple phrases that promote physical (and mental) relaxation. These phrases are:

Autogenic Training Phrases

1. My hands and arms are heavy and warm.
2. My feet and legs are heavy and warm.
3. My heartbeat is calm and regular.
4. My breathing is easy and free.
5. My belly is soft and relaxed.
6. My forehead is cool.

This series of statements is repeated for ten to fifteen minutes. Regularly practicing this simple technique helps normalize autonomic nervous system function, reduces anxiety and depression, improves sleep, and helps manage stress[83]. The Ohio State University's Center for Integrative Health and Wellness provides a free MP3 recording of autogenic training on its website, http://go.osu.edu/guidedimagerypractices.

What Is an Optimal Healing Environment?

Few healers would choose to work in a noisy, dirty, or smelly setting. But just what is optimal in terms of a healing environment?

---

83 Kanji N.A., et al., "Autogenic training to reduce anxiety in nursing students: randomized controlled trial," *J Adv Nurs* 53, no. 6 (2006): 729–35. Stetter F., et al., "Autogenic training: a meta-analysis of clinical outcome studies," *Appl Psychophysiol Biofeedback* 27, no. 1 (2002): 45–98. Goldbeck L., et al., "Effectiveness of autogenic relaxation training on children and adolescents with behavioral and emotional problems," *J Am Acad Child Adolesc Psychiatry* 42, no. 9 (2003): 1046–54.

In 2004, the Samueli Institute held a symposium on Optimal Healing Environments in Health Care. The conference leaders, Drs. Wayne Jonas and Ronald Chez, identified seven components of the optimal healing environment[84]:

Dr. Jonas' Optimal Healing Environment

1. Clear intention, awareness, expectation, and belief that healing is possible
2. Self-care practices that promote a sense of wholeness and well-being
3. Techniques that foster a healing presence of compassion, love, and awareness of interconnectedness
4. Communication and listening skills that promote healthy, respectful relationships
5. Promoting health-sustaining lifestyle behaviors, service, and supportive relationships
6. Use of appropriate therapies and practices to promote healing
7. Optimal physical space—architecture, color, light, music, and other elements that foster well-being.

While you may not always be able to control every element of the environment in which you work, be sure to ask the recipient if the things you can control are optimal—temperature, sounds (music or sounds from nature), aromas (essential oils or no fragrances), light levels (bright/dark) privacy (door open or closed), and furniture/ props (blanket, pillow, or cushions to promote a supported posture

---

84 Jonas W.B. and Chez R.A., "Toward Optimal Healing Environments in Healthcare," *J Alt Comp Med* 10, S1 (2004): S1–S6.

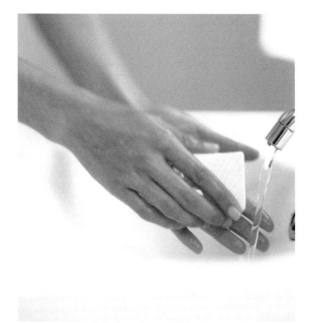

Used with permission from Microsoft

so the recipient can rest comfortably). Most people feel best in a clean, uncluttered room with natural light and a view of nature or natural scenes.

The micro-environment is also important. Wash your hands before and after every healing session.

Does this mean you cannot be of assistance in a less-than-optimal environment? No. Here's an example.

At the departure gate at the airport several years ago, I encountered a colleague and his family who were waiting for the same flight. His daughter had taken a bad turn on some gravel and fell off her rented motorbike the day before.

She ended up in the emergency department with scrapes and bruises over most of the left side of her face and body. Now she was covered in bandages, sitting stiffly in obvious pain with her back to the wall and her left foot propped on a suitcase. When I asked if she'd like me to try something to help her feel more comfortable, she agreed with typical teenage skepticism. I asked my colleague to stand in front of her, and with me on her left side, and her siblings at her right side, she had at least a little privacy. Within a few minutes, she said, "I do feel more comfortable! It's like the pain is melting away!" Her father was dubious. I suggested he hold his hands a few inches over his daughter's scraped shoulder and compare it to the sensation on the unharmed right side of her body. "They're really different! The left side is much hotter," he noted. As we continued the work, the father intermittently compared the left and right sides. When the sides were nearly equal in temperature by his estimate, the daughter's pain had gone from a seven out of ten to a one out of ten. He was amazed. "This is so obvious," he noted. "I had a harder time learning to listen to hearts or look in ears. Why didn't they teach this in medical school?" Indeed, why don't we teach it in medical school, and nursing school, and in physical therapy training?

So, even in an airport departure gate, it is possible to have a healing experience. Being internally prepared allows us to serve others, regardless of the external circumstances. Although we'd rather be able to silence the overhead announcements and play soothing music, view scenes from nature rather than airport runways, and provide cushions rather than a suitcase for support, we can serve when and where we are called, regardless of the surroundings.

What else is helpful in preparing to do healing work? Breathing and visualization practices are extremely helpful. Let's explore them in the next chapter.

CHAPTER 6

Breathing and Imagery Practices

"Feelings come and go like clouds in a windy sky.
Conscious breathing is my anchor."

—THÍCH NHÁT HÁNH

FROM OUR FIRST BREATH as a newborn, to our last breath before death, our breath is our constant companion. We can survive a month without food, a few days without water, but only minutes without breathing. A deliberate focus on slow, deep breaths is part of La-maze preparation for childbirth. When we are stressed, our friends and family may remind us to take a deep breath to help restore our inner peace.

Since ancient times, breathing practices have been an important part of healing. For example, in the Ayurvedic healing practices of India, the science of breathing is known as "pranayama." The breath (prana) is equated with the life force. In Christianity, God breathed the breath of life into the first humans.

When we are relaxed, our breathing slows, and by deliberately slowing our breathing, we can generate a sense of relaxation. In addition, intentional visualization can help promote both centering and grounding. Deliberate attention to the breath and imagination are powerful tools for healers.

Relaxed breathing has a 1:1 ratio of breathing in (inspiration) to breathing out (expiration). When we are relaxed, as we breathe in, first the belly (abdomen) softens and expands, then the lower chest, and finally the upper chest fills out. As we breathe out, contraction occurs in reverse order: upper chest, lower chest, and finally the abdomen. You don't have to force it. Allow the breath to flow in and out naturally, easily, deeply, and rhythmically. It may help to put a hand over your belly so you can feel the relaxed movements of the belly out (as you breathe in) and in (as you breathe out).

Counting Breaths

Counting breaths is a simple way to relax and focus attention. Use the relaxed, rhythmic breathing in these five easy steps.

Counting Breaths in Five Easy Steps

1. Sit, stand, or lay in a comfortable position in which you are supported and relaxed. Become aware of your breathing. Allow your eyes to close or focus on an object a few feet away, such as a candle or peaceful, inspiring image.
2. Count each breath in and out as one cycle, going from 1 to 10.

    For example, I breathe in. I breathe out. 1.

    I breathe in. I breathe out. 2.

    I breathe in. I breathe out. 3.

    And so on, through 10.
3. Repeat. You do not need to force yourself to breathe at a

particular speed or depth. Just continue the counting of breaths in a cycle of 10. If you lose track, return to 1 and start over.

4. When thoughts arise, observe and release them. Return to awareness of the breath and counting.

5. Continue for 10 to 20 minutes. Do not worry about whether you have maintained your focus or your mind has wandered. When you notice your mind wandering, simply return to your focus. You do not have to force a particular outcome. It may help you to relax to set a small timer so you don't have to look at a clock to know when the practice period is up.

This practice not only promotes relaxation, it also builds attention and focus, and helps lower blood pressure in those with hypertension.

Must you count to ten? No. You can simply repeat the word "one" with each breath. Or count to three or seven or whatever your favorite number is. Once you master counting to ten without mind-wandering or losing your place, you can increase the number to twelve, twenty, or fifty to stretch your capacity to focus.

The 4-7-8 Breath

My friend and colleague, Tieraona Low Dog, M.D., recommends the 4-7-8 breath as a great antidote to stress. It has just four steps.

The 4-7-8 Stress-Buster Breath

1. Sit, stand, or lay in a comfortable position in which you are supported and relaxed. Become aware of your breathing.

Allow your eyes to close or focus on an object a few feet away, such as a candle or peaceful, inspiring image.

2. Count each breath in and out as one cycle.

   Breathe in to a count of 4.

   Hold your breath for a count of 7.

   Breathe out to a count of 8.

3. Repeat the cycle four times.

4. When thoughts arise, observe and release them.

Do not worry about whether you have maintained your focus or your mind has wandered.

> *"I took a deep breath and listened to the old brag of my heart.*
> *I am, I am, I am."*
>
> —Sylvia Plath, *The Bell Jar*

Do You Have to Count or Use Numbers?

No. Some people dislike numbers and would rather focus on repeating a word or phrase. This is fine, too. You can simply repeat a positive or neutral word (e.g., "peace" or "one") or phrase (e.g., "I am") with each breath.

> *"When you own your breath, no one can steal your peace."*
>
> —Anonymous

Ocean Breathing

One variation on slow deep breathing is called ocean breathing. In this variation, you don't need to count or focus on a phrase or word.

As with the other practices, you breathe in and out through your nose, slowly and deeply. With the in-breath, first the belly expands, then the lower chest, and finally the upper chest. With the out-breath, the sequence is reversed, so the belly is the last to move inward. The tongue touches the roof of the mouth just behind the top front teeth. On the out-breath, the back of the throat is slightly constricted, so as the air moves out, there is a noise like snoring or the sound of the ocean. This breath promotes relaxation and alertness simultaneously. It sounds a bit odd, so it's best to practice this when alone or in a group with others doing the same practice.

Want Help and Love Technology?

Try a metronome. A metronome is a device many musicians use to set a steady tempo. Both electronic and wind-up models are available; you may also find a metronome app for your smartphone or tablet. Simply set the metronome to 60 beats per minute, and then breathe in to a count of five and out to a count of five. This gives you six breaths per minute. Try slowing to a count of six for each in-breath and out-breath (five breaths per minute). Then try breathing in and out to a count of four (a little faster than seven breaths per minute). Do you notice any difference? Use the rate that seems most comfortable for you. Use this paced breathing approach five to ten minutes once or twice daily. Paced breathing helps lower sympathetic (fight or flight) activity and increases parasympathetic (rest-digest) activity. It can help lower stress.

The RespERate® is an FDA-approved device for lowering blood pressure. The device includes headphones and an elastic belt that fits snugly and comfortably around your chest. Both connect to a central processor unit. The unit measures your breathing rate, and then plays relaxing music with distinct tones to signal the next in-breath and out-breath. The central processor also displays your breathing rate and provides a visual cue to breathe in and out with the tones. At first the signal keeps pace with your breathing, and then it gradually slows. You don't have to count or remember anything other than to breathe with the tones and visual cue (the tones allow you to close your eyes while you practice). This is a good choice for people who are more focused on sound than visual cues. Insurance may cover some of the cost if you have high blood pressure and your doctor writes a note for you.

The Institute of HeartMath offers a biofeedback device (EmWave® Personal Stress Reliever) and software programs (e.g., GPS for the Soul®) that also provide visual signals for slow deep breathing. You can adjust the device to different breathing rates and just follow the bouncing ball or opening and closing flower. As your breathing slows and synchronizes with the signal, you receive feedback that reinforces your practice.

As technology advances, there is an increasing number of smartphone and tablet applications that provide feedback or guidance about slow, deep breathing. Few of them have undergone as much research as the RespERate® and HeartMath® products, but future research may reveal similarities. In the meantime, for those who love new technology and want to try a device to help promote slow, deep breathing, I recommend these products because I have reviewed studies about them, used them myself, and found them helpful.

What If You're Feeling Sluggish and Want to Use the Breath to Feel More Energy?

Breathing practices can be used to energize and increase a sense of vitality as well as to relax. Dr. Andrew Weil suggests the "bellows breath" to get your inner fire going. If you've ever tried to get a dying fire flaming again, you know exactly what this means. It's a rapid breath done for a short period of time. Start with fifteen seconds, and do not exceed one minute[85].

Bellows Breath

1. Be aware of your breath. Put your hand on your belly so you can feel it move out with the in-breath and in with the out-breath.
2. Breathe in and out through your nose as rapidly as possible, aiming for two to three breaths per second.
3. Stop. If you do this for a long period of time, you may get dizzy from hyperventilating and excessively lowering your body's natural carbon dioxide level.

Breathing Together

Human beings are finely tuned social beings. We tend to mirror each other's patterns of speech, mannerisms, and even breathing patterns. As you become aware of this kind of mutual influence, you will want to become more mindful of being an influence for positive, peaceful breathing patterns.

One of the quickest ways to establish rapport and empathy is to breathe together. As the recipient is talking or resting, simply observe his breathing, and synchronize your breathing with him. Stay together for three to four breaths, and be aware of breathing slightly louder than usual (but not so loud that it's creepy) so it's easier for the recipient,

---

85 Breathing fast while at rest for several minutes can lead to very low carbon dioxide levels (hyperventilation) and a feeling of panic and light-headedness. Please do not exceed one minute of this exercise. And if you are prone to anxiety or panic attacks, you may want to skip it altogether.

especially if his eyes are closed, to be aware of your breathing. Then gradually slow your breathing. The recipient is likely to follow your new, slower pace, gradually relaxing as his breathing slows.

It is easier to breathe together intentionally when you are both silent than it is when you are in the middle of a conversation. Try it the next time you are relaxing with a loved one listening to music or watching a movie, or with a colleague while you are both listening during a meeting, or with a stranger while you're waiting in line. This is a great exercise for becoming more aware of and focused on subtle cues such as breathing patterns.

Breathing Visualizations

The breath not only helps us obtain and circulate oxygen, it also helps rid us of carbon dioxide and other wastes and toxins. If you've ever eaten raw garlic, you know that you soon exhale pungent fumes. This means that in addition to getting rid of carbon dioxide, the lungs can expel other volatile (gassy or vaporous) compounds that drift through the thin membranes in the lungs separating the blood from the breath. Remember that the carbon dioxide we exhale is actually nourishing to plants, just as the compost from our kitchen waste is also healthful for plants. In turn, plants "exhale" oxygen, which is vital to us.

Many people use visualization along with deep, rhythmic, relaxed breathing to further focus attention and calmly center the mind or deepen grounding in the intention to be helpful.

Visualizing the Cleansing Breath

1. Sit or rest in a safe, relaxed place where you are comfortable and supported.

2. Breathe in, imagining cool, fresh, cleansing, air that fills your lungs with nourishing oxygen.

3. Breathe out, imagining all the used air, toxins, and carbon dioxide naturally flowing outward to the nearest tree or other plant, which will use our waste to create more oxygen.

4. Repeat this cycle as long as you like, repeatedly filling your lungs with cleansing oxygen-rich air that circulates throughout the body, cleansing every organ and tissue, and releasing all the unnecessary compounds back to the earth and plants that use those compounds to nourish us with oxygen and beauty.

We all know our hearts serve as pumps to move blood throughout our body. We can also imagine our diaphragm (the breathing muscle that separates chest from abdomen) as a giant pump, moving air and healing vitality throughout our body and connecting us with nature and other humans.

Breathing in through Your Head, and out through Your Feet

One of the easiest visualization practices is to imagine universal healing energy as a clear light that surrounds and fills you. For this practice, instead of imagining the cleansing breath flowing in and out through your lungs, which is physiologically accurate, we use our imaginations to visualize the diaphragm pulling in healing energy from the top of our heads with the in-breath, and then moving it three different ways with the out-breath—a) circulating throughout the body; b) seeing it flow down and out through the soles of our feet; and c) seeing it flow down and out through the palms of the hands.

Breathing Visualizations

1. Before you begin, set a positive intention for the practice (e.g., healing, relaxing, or learning from the experience).
2. Imagine you are sitting in a quiet, sacred place, like a grove of trees or a cathedral with a beam of light shining down on you. This light is cleansing, protective, and allows you to relax deeply.
3. As you breathe in, imagine your diaphragm, heart, and lungs drawing this universal, inspiring, healing light in through the top of your head, through your brain, your throat, your upper chest and arms, down into your heart and lungs. In your heart, the universal healing light mixes with your compassionate intention. Remember, your heart/lungs are pumps, drawing the light-energy in, mixing it, and then gently circulating it.
4. As you breathe out, imagine the diaphragm, heart, and lungs *circulating the healing light energy throughout your body*, protecting, cleansing, restoring, balancing, revitalizing, and harmonizing as needed. Draw in another breath; circulate again. Repeat several times.
5. When you have circulated the healing energy several times, you are ready to redirect it downward and *out through the feet*. On your next breath, after you breathe in and mix the universal healing energy with your heart's pure intention, imagine your diaphragm, lungs, and heart gently pumping the healing energy down from your heart, through your solar plexus and lower abdomen, down your legs, and out your toes or the soles of your feet. If you like, you can imagine the energy flowing in through your brain, down your spinal cord, and out through your feet, aided by the large set of pumps in the

middle of your chest. Repeat several times. This is sometimes called the Middle Pillar visualization—the core of your body in front of your backbone is the middle pillar along which you can imagine the light-energy flowing from top to bottom[86].

Optional imagery practice: *out of the hands*. After you breathe in the universal healing light-energy and it mixes with your pure heart-centered intention, as you breathe out, imagine the healing energy being pumped from your lungs and heart, down your harms, through your hands, flowing just where it's needed. Notice how your hands feel after several out-breaths of healing light-energy have flowed through them.

Optional imagery practice: *working with colors*. See what this breathing and visualization experience is like for you if you imagine the universal healing energy as a clear white, blue, green, or golden light. These are the most commonly used healing colors; most healers recommend avoiding colors like black, gray, brown, or muddy tones. Stay with one color for several breaths. What do you notice?

Breathing in white or clear light through the top of the head and out through the feet usually leads to a sense of cleansing and protection, leading to relaxation. Visualizing a deep cobalt blue can deepen a sense of relaxation. But what if you're already relaxed and want to feel stronger and more revitalized?

Breathing in through Your Feet and out through Your Hands

Once you have mastered the imagery of breathing in universal healing light energy from the top of your head and out through your feet

---

86 Israel Regardie and Marc Allen, *The Art of True Healing: the unlimited power of prayer and visualization*, (New World Library, 1932 reprinted in 1997).

or hands, you can learn to imagine that the nurturing, strengthening, supportive, revitalizing energy of Mother Earth is flowing into your feet and up into your core with each breath in.

Breathing to Circulate Earth Energy through Hands

1. Before you begin, set an intention (e.g., healing, revitalization, or learning).
2. Imagine that Mother Earth is filled with healing energy, strength, and vitality.
3. As you breathe in, draw up this nurturing, practical, revitalizing healing energy through the soles of your feet, up through the marrow of your bones into your heart. In your heart, Mother Earth's healing energy is joined to your compassionate intention.
4. As you breathe out, imagine this strong, nurturing earth energy *circulating throughout your body*, restoring, balancing, revitalizing, and harmonizing as needed. Repeat for several breaths until you feel ready for the next step, or you can stop here and rest.
5. Continue breathing the revitalizing Mother Earth energy in through your feet, up through your legs, belly, and to your heart, mixing with your positive intention, and then flowing on the *out-breath* down your arms, through your hands, flowing just where it's needed.
6. Continue for as long as you like. Feel gratitude to Mother Earth and yourself for this time together.

Alternating In-Breath through the Head and through the Feet

After you've done both of these breathing practices, imagining breathing in through your head and imagining breathing in through your feet, you can combine them, alternating breaths. Personally, this is one of my favorite practices, as it gives me a strong sense of being centered between the Mother Earth and the Father Sky, between the power of clarity and protection and the power of nurturing practicality in the earth.

Earth–Sky Breathing Combination

1. Set an intention for the practice: healing, learning, relaxing, connecting, increasing vitality, or whatever you choose.
2. On breath one (and subsequent odd-number breaths), as you inhale, imagine drawing in universal, sacred, purifying, protecting, clarifying, and calming healing energy through the top of the head, down into the heart. As you exhale, circulate or move the energy through your body, out through your hands, or out through your feet, whichever suits your current intention.
3. On breath two (and subsequent even number breaths), as you inhale, draw in Mother Earth's revitalizing energy through the soles of your feet, up through your shinbones, thigh bones, pelvis and hip bones, and back bone to your heart. As you exhale, circulate the strong compassionate healing energy out your hands.
4. Repeat the cycle of breath one and breath two, alternately drawing from the healing energy of the universe (sky) and the earth for several minutes.

5. Now relax and breathe normally. What do you notice about how you feel?

Breathing in Comfort; Breathing out Discomfort

If you are experiencing pain in a specific part of your body, you can use your breathing/imagination to achieve a greater sense of comfort and ease.

Breathing for Comfort

1. Identify the area you'd like to feel better.
2. As you breathe in, breathe the healing light energy directly into that area. Or if you prefer, you can breathe in through the top of your head or the soles of your feet and direct the healing energy into the area in need of healing.
3. In the pause between breathing in and out, imagine the healing energy comforting the area of need.
4. As you breathe out, imagine the discomfort leaving the area, leaving the healing light and energy to remain and restore healthy function and sensation.
5. Repeat as needed.

We often find that as we may move attention to an area, the sensations there change. The next time you notice an ache, pain, cramp, or discomfort, rather than distracting yourself by ignoring it or focusing on something else, notice what happens if you go right to the middle of it. Try to find the spot where it is most intense. What are its characteristics? How far out does it extend? Does the quality change with distance from the center? Is it associated with a temperature, color, or sound? How does it change as you breathe into this area and release the sensations on the out-breath? What happens if you put your hand over the area as you breathe in and out of it? Maintain a sense of neutral, friendly curiosity to your experience and notice the changes.

Throughout history, healers have combined visualizations like these with breathing exercises to develop their sense of being centered and grounded, and to increase their awareness of subtle energy flows in their bodies[87]. Commonly identified circuits, such as the traditional acupuncture meridians and energy hubs like the Ayurvedic chakras, are discussed at greater length in Chapter 10.

It is tempting to delve into a variety of visualization practices, but for now, let's simply summarize the purpose of combining breathing and visualization practices: healing. Generally, our healing intentions are one or more of these three: a) promote relaxation and stress reduction; b) promote a greater sense of vitality and energy; and/ or c) relieve suffering or pain by increasing a sense of comfort and ease. By learning to modulate your own relaxation, comfort, and energy levels with the simple techniques described here, you are well on your way to helping others achieve their goals, as well.

Summary of Breathing Practices

Before going into specific healing techniques, let's do just a bit more preparation to ensure we have a firm foundation. This will help us avoid the dragons of fantasy and wishful thinking. The tips in the next two chapters provide a fantastic foundation for emotional and mental preparation for healing work.

---

87 Fascinating visualization exercises are described in Penney Peirce's book, *Frequency: the Power of Personal Vibration*, (New York: Simon and Schuster, 2009) and Keith Sherwood's, *The Art of Spiritual Healing*. (St. Paul: Llewellyn Publications, 2000).

Technique	Purpose/ Description
Counting Breaths	Build relaxation and attention by counting each breath up to 10 and repeating the cycle for 10 to 20 minutes.
4-7-8 Breath	Stress relief. Breathe in to a count of 4; hold it for count of 7; exhale to count of 8; repeat 4 to 5 times.
Ocean Breathing	Build relaxed alertness. Breathing out, constrict the back the throat to make a sound like the ocean as you exhale.
Paced Breathing	Relaxation. Use a metronome set at 60 and breathe in 5 and out 5 steadily. OR use the RespERate™ or EmWave PSR™ device.
Bellows Breath	Energize and build vitality. Rapid shallow breathing for 15 seconds.
Synchronized Breathing	Build empathy. Breathe with a partner or recipient for several minutes, gradually slowing the pace of breathing to 5 to 7 breaths per minutes.
Cleansing Breath	When breathing out, imagine exhaling all toxins, discomfort, and carbon dioxide toward nearest tree, which will take it in and turn it to healthy, healing oxygen.
Breathing in through Head and out through the Hands or Feet	Use your imagination to draw cleansing, power, protection, and nurturing from the universe while maintaining your connection to the earth.
Breathing in through Feet and out through Hands	Use your imagination to draw on Mother Earth's vitality and strength and increase awareness of the sensations of the hands.
Breathing in Comfort/out Discomfort	Enhance a sense of comfort by breathing a sense of healing ease into any uncomfortable areas and allowing the discomfort to flow out through the feet as you exhale.

CHAPTER 7
Emotional Preparation

*"First, remove the plank from your own eye before tackling
the splinter in your brother's eye."*

—Matthew 7:5

"Put your own oxygen mask on before assisting others."

—Flight attendant

Before we begin to help relieve others' stress and suffering, it's wise to get our own emotional and mental lives in order. Working with people who are suffering can be stressful, particularly if we're so empathetic we are prone to picking up others' negative emotions. To be a successful healer over the long term, it behooves us to cultivate emotional and mental stability.

Just as we assume that health professionals will need to study hard to assimilate the knowledge and skills necessary for being successful professionals, shouldn't we also expect to do a little work to ensure we are emotionally and mentally ready to tackle the challenges of working with suffering?

Although most of us think of emotions as things that automatically happen outside of our control, we can activate neutral and positive or desirable emotions intentionally. The more often we activate positive emotions, the easier it is to access and use them for healing. On the other hand, the more we dwell in and linger on the negative emotions, the more we get in our own way of being effective. Can we completely avoid negative emotions? Not if we're human! We cannot avoid negative emotions any more than we can avoid becoming hungry or tired, but we can recognize the thought or emotion and respond appropriately to minimize their adverse impact on ourselves and others.

Emotions Table

Desirable Emotions and Attitudes	Negative or Afflictive Emotions
Appreciation, gratitude	Envy
Caring, compassion, kindness, love, affection	Pride, vanity
Peace, calm, serenity, contentment	Anxiety, fear
Harmony, balance, connectedness	Anger, rage
Confidence, courage	Lethargy, sloth, laziness
Joy, happiness, delight, gladness, pleasure, good cheer, satisfaction	Self-pity
Anticipation, hope, optimism	Greed
Ecstasy, exhilaration, bliss, exultation	Depression

Think about the list. Imagine feeling one or more of these positive emotions. Do you remember the last time you really felt this way? What was happening? Where were you? Who was with you? What were you doing? What did you see, hear, smell, and feel?

When we vividly recall strong emotions, our bodies respond just as if we were actually there. When you activate a positive emotion, your body relaxes; your hormones and neurotransmitter production, heart rate, breathing, and blood pressure all shift into a more positive mode; and your mind becomes more focused and clear. This can help you become a more effective healer.

The first step in managing your emotions is to *recognize your current emotion*. Sometimes just recognizing your current emotion helps shift it. Do not condemn the emotion. You wouldn't condemn your body for letting you know it's hungry or thirsty; why get upset with it when it's giving you an emotional signal? The next time you notice that you are feeling sad, angry, or envious, turn to that emotion with gentle, friendly curiosity. Can you notice when the emotion began, or has it been there a while, quietly escalating until its presence was shouting? Where in your body do you feel it the most? Do you feel a sense of heat or cold, tightness or relaxation? Try imagining yourself sitting in a movie theater watching yourself sitting a few rows in front of you, watching yourself on the giant screen. Cultivate the sense of being an interested observer, extending goodwill and kindness toward yourself.

Simply shifting to neutral may be enough. Being aware of what you are feeling and thinking, and observing thoughts, emotions, and sensations with kind curiosity as they change over time is called *mindfulness* or *insight*. Numerous studies have shown that practicing mindful, insightful awareness can be a powerful antidote to depression, anxiety, and stress.

This is an important skill for healers. However, it may not be sufficient to generate the kind of positive energy you want to uplift another person who is suffering. With practice, it is possible to shift, not just from negative to neutral, but from neutral to a positive emotional state.

To shift toward the positive state, we don't combat the negative or neutral state, make it wrong, or ignore it, but we shift our attention and imagination toward our goal. To do this, it helps to have a *concrete image* of the *desired* emotion, not just an abstract idea. Let's say you want to practice engendering the feeling "contentment." For most people, focusing on an actual experience is likely to be more effective than just focusing on the word "contentment."

For example, imagine how you feel when you pet a dog (assuming you've petted a dog and liked it), or imagine sitting in a beautiful place with loved ones following a delicious meal. Conjure up the visual image, sound, tactile feelings, smells, and internal bodily sensations associated with that experience of contentment. Savor it.

One of the most reliable, easily achieved, and helpful emotions to practice is *appreciation* or gratitude. This practice is so effective as a stress management tool that the Institute of HeartMath has built an entire emotional self-management training program around it[88].

Practice Gratitude

Before you start this emotional self-management practice, make a list of the people, experiences, places, events, or things for which you *genuinely* feel grateful. For example, I truly appreciate:

- *People and pets:* my family, my teachers, students, patients, friends, neighbors, cats, the men who take my garbage away every week, the mail delivery person, the grocery store clerk who smiles at me, the person who held the elevator for me
- *Events/circumstances:* having hot running water when I turn on the shower; having electricity when I plug in the computer; flowers that bloom by the side of the road

---

88 McCraty, R., et al,. "The impact of an emotional self-management skills course on psychosocial functioning and autonomic recovery to stress in middle school children," *Integr Physiol Behav Sci* 34, no. 4 (1999): 246–68.

- *Things:* home, safe transportation, waterfalls in the mountains, favorite bookstore, favorite warm sweater when it is cold, a car that starts, public transportation that arrives on time, safely, and at a reasonable price

None of these things needs to be perfect. Focus on the positive aspects that you truly, deeply, genuinely appreciate. Make your own list. You don't have to break it into categories. Just jot down three things you appreciate.

I truly appreciate (or I am grateful for):

1. _____

2. _____

3. _____

It's okay if you start with a short list, and it's okay to change your list. The important thing is that you have at least *one* thing on your list for which you truly feel grateful.

Practicing Gratitude

Now that you have a list, here's the practice.

A. Focus on a part of your *body* that feels neutral or comfortable. Focusing on your body helps you embody the practice and make it less abstract. Positive emotions generate real effects on the body, including the brain. For most people, it's easiest to focus on the center of your forehead, chest, or belly, just below your belly button, wherever is comfortable or neutral for you. Got it? Good.

B. Notice your *breathing.* Just allow it to be smooth, regular, and even. You don't need to force it. You don't need to breathe a particular way. You can breathe through your nose or mouth. Being aware of your breathing helps connect you with your current life, right now, in this moment. You are breathing in and out. You are alive. Just let it be smooth and even, relaxed and easy.

C. While aware of your body and breath, *choose* that feeling of gratitude. Just think about that person, pet, event, circumstance, place, or thing. It's okay to let your mind wander to other things for which you feel truly grateful. However, for this practice time, if you notice that your mind starts to wander to a worry, a conflict, something sad, what you need to do later, or what you should have said, just notice that and return to your focus on gratitude. You can get to that other thing in just a little while. It can wait a few minutes, and in fact, your mind will be clearer and better able to address that situation after you've finished this practice. Maintain your focus for your chosen length of time.

D. When you have finished your appreciation practice for the length of time you chose, *congratulate* yourself on practicing something that helps you become a more effective healer. When would you like to practice again? Consider practicing several times a day. Do it again.

That's it. Remember to focus on a neutral part of your body; take slow, relaxing breaths; focus on appreciation; celebrate your successful practice; and plan to do it again. If you'd like additional coaching on this technique, look for a HeartMath certified trainer.

Benefits of Gratitude

Intentionally activating a feeling of gratitude has many benefits. Physiologically, it helps lower cortisol (a stress hormone) while enhancing the coherent, harmonious function of the autonomic nervous system[89]; it helps lower high blood pressure[90]; and it lowers levels of stress hormones, such as cortisol[91]. Gratitude helps your mind function with greater clarity and improves your mood[92]. Intentional practice helps you achieve a sense of mastery and control, improves insight and problem-solving abilities, and decreases anxiety[93]. You may not be able to affect whether the sun comes up tomorrow or how other people behave, but you can choose to be aware of your body, mindfully breathe, and practice a positive emotion for ten seconds. Practicing one positive emotion readies your brain and heart for easier access to other positive emotions. The more you practice, the more proficient you become.

Here is a model or map for the relationships between positive and negative emotions of high or low intensity:

Emotional Map

On the emotional map, the north and south poles are high and low intensity, while the east and west directions point to positive and negative emotions.

---

89 McCraty R., et al., "The effect of emotions on short-term power spectrum analysis of heart rate variability," *Am J Cardiol* 76, no. 14 (1995): 1089–93.

90 McCraty R., et al., "Impact of a workplace stress reduction program on blood pressure and emotional health in hypertensive employees," *J Altern Complement Med* 9, no. 3 (2003): 355–69.

91 McCraty R., et al., "The impact of a new emotional self-management program on stress, emotions, heart rate variability, DHEA, and cortisol," *Integr Physiol Behav Sci* 33, no. 2 (1998): 151–70.

92 Fredrickson B.L., et al., "Open hearts build lives: positive emotions, induced through loving-kindness meditation, build consequential personal resources," *J Pers Soc Psychol* 95, no. 5 (2008): 1042–62.

93 Subramaniam K., et al., "A brain mechanism for facilitation of insight by positive affect," *J Cogn Neurosci* 21, no. 3 (2009): 415–32.

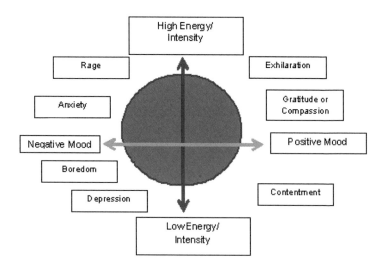

Warm Up with Gratitude

You can also warm up for a healing session by practicing gratitude before you start. Just focus on your body, breathe, and feel grateful for something. After a brief gratitude warm-up, you may find it easier to communicate more effectively and pleasantly than you'd anticipated. And you may also find it easier to be centered and grounded while becoming more observant of the person you are helping.

Practice Gratitude: Journals and More

A *gratitude journal* helps bolster your awareness and builds multiple brain circuits so it's easier to access positive emotions in the future. Keeping a gratitude journal is like putting money in your emotional bank account.

Do's and Don'ts of Keeping a Gratitude Journal

- Don't write the same thing every day (humans habituate quickly).

- Don't worry about spelling, punctuation, or grammar.
- **Do** pay attention throughout the day to what you might include.
- **Do** make the conscious decision to use this experience to enrich your life, build your happiness, and help you become more positive.
- **Do** write in it at least one to three times per week.
- **Do** focus on elaborating in depth on a few items rather than listing many things superficially. Consider expanding a bit on "why" the good thing happened.
- **Do** focus on personal gratitude (what someone did for you) rather than simply material gratitude (what you have).
- **Do** include unexpected or surprise sources of gratitude. This promotes a sense of delight and joy as well as gratitude.
- **Do** share your gratitude with others. Sharing positive experiences increases the positive emotion associated with it, and events that are shared are more likely to be remembered.

Speaking of journals, writing regularly about daily experiences is another effective strategy for boosting well-being. As we write about an event, we gain a new perspective and a little distance, allowing us to see things more objectively and clearly. Writing your most meaningful experiences down can help you process them, and improve your mood and memory[94]. Writers have many choices in how to write about what happened, and considering these choices increases the sense of autonomy—the power to choose. Strengthening

94 Klein K., et al., "Expressive writing can increase working memory capacity," *J Exp Psychol Gen* 130, no. 3 (2001): 520–33. Lepore S.J., "Expressive writing moderates the relation between intrusive thoughts and depressive symptoms," *J Pers Soc Psychol* 73, no. 5 (1997): 1030–7.

a sense of autonomy is an excellent way to improve mental and emotional resilience.

If you don't want to jot in a journal, you have other options. Talk into a recorder, post to social media, or tell a friend or family member. Telling your family, friends, and colleagues how much you appreciate them is a great way to improve morale and prevent burnout[95]. Another useful practice is to write thank you notes. Or begin and end email messages with a phrase of gratitude: "Thanks for writing"; "Thanks for taking the time to . . ."; "Thanks for collaborating . . ."; "Thanks for alerting me to this situation"; "Thanks for your" . . . candor, insight, or timeliness.

Another useful practice to generate and share gratitude is saying thanks before meals. Thanks for the food, those who grew it, brought it to you, prepared it, served it, made it possible for you to have it. Or take turns expressing gratitude for something that happened with those sharing the meal with you.

Note the simple things that really enrich your life[96]. It could be the taste of a fresh strawberry, the hug of a child, the presence of a pet, the sun, or the rain.

Practicing gratitude sounds very simple. It is actually a very ancient practice. It's even older than my grandmother, who told me that the secret to overcoming worry and falling asleep easily was to "count your blessings." The more you practice feeling grateful, the easier it gets. Modern science supports this ancient wisdom[97].

---

95 White, P.E., "Unhappy? Low morale? Try the 5 languages of appreciation in the workplace," *J Christ Nurs* 29, no. 3 (2012): 144–9.

96 Lyubomirsky S.L., et al., "The costs and benefits of writing, talking, and thinking about life's triumphs and defeats. *J Pers Soc Psychol* 90, number 4 (2006): 692–708.

97 Emmons R.A., et al., "Counting blessings versus burdens: an experimental investigation of gratitude and subjective well-being in daily life," *J Pers Soc Psychol* 84, no. 2 (2003): 377–89. Kashdan T.B., et al., "Gratitude and hedonic and eudaimonic well-being in Vietnam war veterans," *Behav Res Ther* 44, no. 2 (2006): 177–99.

And here's a side benefit. The more you practice feeling grateful, the more you'll notice there are things to be grateful for, even in situations that used to drive you crazy. Before I started consciously practicing gratitude, I hated to wait at red lights. Now I notice that this red light has given me another minute to practice feeling grateful. There are people whose only job in life is to help me and other drivers get where we are going safely, and it took a lot of them to invent, design, manufacture, install, and maintain this light. Isn't that amazing? There are other drivers who are stopped here, too. Isn't it great that other people follow the rules so we can travel safely? Now that I think about it, I'm very grateful to have a place to go and a way to get there. Red lights? What a blessing!

You might notice that the more you practice gratitude, the more often you naturally feel grateful, even when you aren't even trying. And the more creatively and positively you will see situations, people, and events that may not have seemed so positive in the past. Don't expect to overturn decades of resentment, fear, envy, or disappointment immediately. Be patient with yourself. You'll be amazed at how many benefits you feel the more you practice.

You can use the same simple steps to practice different positive emotions. For example, parents want their children to be happy. Pet owners feel deep affection toward their pet. Doctors and nurses want their patients to feel comfortable, strong, and resilient. Ministers, rabbis, and other spiritual leaders want people to experience peace and connection with a higher power. It's natural to focus on feelings of compassion, kindness, forgiveness, and genuine caring.

Two other helpful emotions to practice are *caring* (affection, loving-kindness, or compassion) and *hope* or *positive anticipation*. You could also practice feeling *confident* or *courageous*, vividly remembering previous experiences in which you've been courageous or when you've accomplished a goal or objective (such as riding a two-wheeled bike without training wheels).

Practice Empathy, Compassion, and Mentally Extending Goodwill

First, some simple definitions:

Empathy: understanding another person's emotional state

Compassion: understanding someone's suffering and desiring to relieve it

Loving-kindness: extending goodwill and kind-hearted best wishes for someone to enjoy and love life.

Empathy

Your goal is to maintain your own emotional well-being while connecting with and understanding someone else. You want her to feel heard, understood, respected, and cared for. You don't want to start suffering with her. So take a deep breath and center before you begin.

The best way to know whether you have understood another accurately is to ask. For example, if you think John is anxious or scared, you might say, "John, it sounds like you are feeling worried; is that right?" If he nods yes, ask if there's anything else. He might answer, "Yes, I'm worried the pain will get worse and that nothing will really help, and I'll never get better." Nod or indicate that you've heard, and ask if there's anything else.

When you think you've got it, repeat it back using your own words and ask if that's correct. If it is, you can say something about how you are here with him to help him feel better, and you are confident that together you can get through this situation. Most people feel a great sense of relief just knowing that someone else understands their situation and they are not alone. And you will feel better knowing you were able to help.

If you can maintain your own emotional well-being, feeling a sense of calm, focus, affection, and compassion while listening, understanding, and connecting, you've done a lot to help. You've already started to help just by listening without trying to judge, interpret, explain, or solve problems. You've avoided the verbal traps that could make someone feel misunderstood, pitied, blamed, stupid, or incompetent.

Experiencing empathy can help you connect with another person and increase your sensitivity and intuition, but it can also leave you feeling exhausted, drained, sad, or irritable if you start to adopt and experience others' suffering chronically. Empathy without compassion and loving-kindness can lead to burnout.

Remember Jets

If you notice that someone is suffering, you may notice that you start to feel uncomfortable, worried, or angry. It is natural to feel bad when someone else is suffering. Before plunging into desperate efforts to cheer or encourage someone else, remember airplanes. First, put on your own mask (become calm and centered) before helping others. If you are tense, angry, or worried, you will be less effective in helping someone else than if you are calm, clear, and focused. Be aware of your body; breathe in, breathe out, and internally be grateful, just for a moment. You might be grateful that you are breathing, grateful that they trust you to be with them, grateful that your heart is beating, grateful for your teachers, or grateful to be alive. Centering and nourishing your own emotional state will allow you to help your loved one more effectively, efficiently, and easily.

Compassion

Moving from empathy to compassion is empowering and strengthens your core because it deepens your grounding. You remember who you are and why you are here, and you take steps to relieve suffering rather than stopping with simply recognizing it. The steps in deepening your practicing compassion are the same as for gratitude.

Compassion Practice

1. Focus on a part of your body, such as the center of your forehead, chest, or belly. This affects you physically, emotionally, and mentally. Be here, in your body, now.
2. Be aware of your *breathing*. Right now, in this moment, you are alive.
3. Intentionally choose a sense of *affection* or *compassion* for a person, pet, circumstance, place, or thing. Imagine this sensation of compassion vividly—how does it look, sound, feel in your body? Sustain it as long as you like. (As with gratitude, you can write a list, keep a journal, create a poem, sing a song, send a message, or just feel it in your heart.)
4. *Congratulate* yourself on practicing and *plan* to do it again.

Scientific studies of practitioners of compassion-based meditation have shown important improvements in the function of several regions of the brain; these brain changes include areas involved in modulating stress responses[98].

---

98 Lutz A., et al., "Regulation of the neural circuitry of emotion by compassion meditation: effects of meditative expertise," *PLoS ONE* 3, no. 3 (2008): e1897.

What Is the Difference between Self-Compassion, Self-Pity, Self-Esteem, and Loving-Kindness?

Self-compassion is not the same as having self-pity or being self-indulgent. It also differs from self-esteem. Both self-pity and self-esteem tend to isolate or separate us from others, whereas self-compassion and loving-kindness tend to help us realize our common humanity with others. Self-compassion allows us to see ourselves more clearly, with neither shame nor arrogance, and it empowers us to take action to relieve suffering. With self-compassion, we see

Self-Compassion	Self-Pity	Self-Esteem	Loving-Kindness
Recognizing that suffering is part of the human condition and trying to relieve it. Sense of common humanity. (Yes, I'm feeling bad, but so are many others, some of whom are worse off than me.) Recognizing one's problems with insight, kindness, and responsibility, without shame or self-condemnation. Knowing that all humans deserve compassion and understanding, not just those with a certain set of traits.	Feeling that you are separate from, and worse off than, others. Forgetting that others have similar problems. Ego-centric separation from others, exaggerating one's personal suffering. Isolating, often leads to self-indulgence (I feel bad, so I'll eat ice cream and watch TV all day).	Feeling better than others; it may lead to self-absorption or narcissism. It can lead to putting down others to feel better about ourselves or ignoring/distorting /hiding our perceived flaws to avoid a sense of shame or inadequacy. May include anger with others who do not recognize our superiority. Self-esteem fluctuates depending on circumstances.	Recognizing that wanting to be safe, healthy, happy, free, and peaceful is part of the human condition, and trying to help yourself and others achieve those goals.

how we are connected to one another. Self-compassion is closely related to loving-kindness, because loving-kindness also acknowledges that all people want to feel safe, secure, healthy, happy, and free. Both loving-kindness and compassion tend to connect us with others, whereas self-pity and self-esteem can both increase a sense of isolation.

Self-Compassion

In our zeal for helping others, it's easy to forget to take care of ourselves, but it is important to offer the same kindness and compassion toward ourselves that we offer clients or patients. Do you tend to be a self-critical perfectionist? Don't worry. Dr. Kristin Neff and her colleagues at the University of Texas have shown that it is possible to set aside that self-critical voice and increase our self-compassion[99]. Practicing self-compassion is a wonderful way to begin the practicing of extending loving-kindness and compassion to everyone.

Here are the four simple phrases I repeat for this practice. I pair one phrase or sentence with one breath. So the entire practice takes four breaths, which can be repeated for several minutes:

Self-Compassion Practice
1. May I be safe and secure.
2. May I be healthy, comfortable, and at ease.
3. May I be happy and peaceful.
4. May I be free from suffering and its causes.

---

99 Neff K.D. and Germer C.K., "A pilot study and randomized controlled trial of the mindful self-compassion program," *J Clin Psychol* 69, no. 1 (2013): 28–44.

You can substitute a positive phrase of your choice. One little boy who learned this practice decided to include: "May I be wild and free!" Choose phrases that bring you a sense of contentment, joy, and liberation.

Research shows that practicing compassion and loving-kindness toward self and others leads to greater happiness and decreased worry[100].

Extending Goodwill or Loving-Kindness

Extending goodwill helps you feel more expansive and open. It helps you affirm a belief that good things can exist. Sincere goodwill is an excellent antidote to feeling jealous.

Here are the four simple phrases I use for this practice. Pair one phrase or sentence with one breath. So the entire practice takes four breaths, which can be repeated for several minutes:

Extending Goodwill or Loving-Kindness
1. May you be safe and secure.
2. May you be healthy, comfortable, and at ease.
3. May you be happy and peaceful.
4. May you be free from suffering and its causes.

You can modify this sequence as you wish. For example, you could substitute, "May all children be safe and secure." Or "May all elderly people be healthy and filled with vitality," or "May all those who mourn find comfort," or "May all those who are lonely experience

---

100 Jazaieri H., et al., "A randomized controlled trial of compassion cultivation training: effects on mindfulness, affect, and emotion regulation," *Motivation and Emotion* 38, no. 1 (2014): 23–35.

love and support," or "May all those living in war zones experience peace and security," or "May all those who are hungry be fed."

Summary of Emotional Preparation Practices

Practice	Purpose and Summary
Recognize current emotion	Increase self-awareness and mindfulness. Recognize emotional state with kind curiosity. Avoid self-criticism or self-judgment.
Engender a positive emotion	Build emotional self-regulatory skills. Focus on all the senses associated with experiencing a positive emotion.
Gratitude meditation	Build a specific positive emotion to enhance emotional capacity. Focus on a neutral part of the body; notice breathing; reflect on gratitude. OR reflect on gratitude prior to an anticipated challenge. Or keep a gratitude journal OR give thanks before meals OR write thank you notes.
Empathy- building	Enhance awareness of others' emotional states. Ask; reflect; ask for correction. Avoid trying to "fix" or change another's emotional state. Seek to understand and support rather than change.
Compassion and loving-kindness meditation	Build a specific positive emotion to enhance emotional capacity. Focus on a neutral part of the body; notice breathing; reflect on someone for whom you care and wish well (including self): May you/I be safe and secure. May you/I be healthy, comfortable, and at ease. May you/I be happy and peaceful. May you/I be free from suffering and its causes.

Practicing emotional self-regulation and intentionally moving to neutral or positive emotions are important strategies to prepare for healing work. They help us slow down and center, re-setting our autonomic nervous system toward "calm" and our brains toward "effective problem-solving[101]." It's also important to prepare mentally and spiritually. That's what the next two chapters are about.

---

101 Brown K.W., "Self-compassion training modulates alpha-amylase, heart rate variability, and subjective responses to social evaluative threat in women," *Psychoneuroendocrinology* 42 (2014): 49–58. May C.J., et al., "Short-term training in loving-kindness meditation produces a state, but not a trait, alteration of attention," *Mindfulness* (April 2011).

CHAPTER 8
Mental Readiness

IN ADDITION TO PHYSICAL AND EMOTIONAL PREPARATION, you can use *mental* practices to promote centering and grounding to prepare for healing. Mental practices or exercises share the generic name of meditation (mental training). The word *meditation* comes from the same root as the word *medicine*. Both historical experience and modern science suggest that meditation has important benefits when practiced regularly.

The two main types of meditation are:

Concentration or focused attention: a conscious focus on a desired intention, object, word, phrase, sound, or image; returning to the intended focus when the mind wanders

Mindfulness: intentional, curious, friendly, warm-hearted non-judgmental awareness of and insight into the ever-changing milieu of current experiences, thoughts, sensations, and emotions.

Both kinds of meditation offer healers a stronger sense of well-being and inner tranquility, less anxiety, and better concentration. I recommend that healers learn and practice both types. You may find that one is easier than another. Embrace the paradox of remaining centered and grounded while extending your awareness, sensitivity, and compassion to yourself and others.

The rest of this chapter provides simple guidance for meditation. Meditation directions sound simple, but the challenge lies in the actual practice. As soon as we try to meditate, we find our minds wandering or judgments arise. On average, it takes less than eight seconds for our minds to wander to something else. This is normal. The key to successful practice is to notice when it happens and then to gently return our awareness to the original intention. There are a number of excellent books, CDs, DVDs, MP3 files, apps for smart devices, YouTube videos on meditation, and electronic courses available online (See the Ohio State University online course on Mind-Body Skills Training for Resilience, Effectiveness, and Mindfulness, http://mind-bodyhealth.osu.edu which lists resources). Additional help from a teacher, coach, or counselor, or practice group can be very useful.

Concentration-Based or Focused-Attention Meditation

What are possible objects of intentional attention? Some people focus on a physical object, such as a candle, a sound, or word. Some people focus on an activity like breathing, or a part of the body, like the heart or space between the eyebrows or the tip of the nose. Find a practice that suits you, and practice regularly to develop a deep sense of its benefits for improving attention and the meta-cognitive skill of being aware of your awareness.

One of the most common types of concentration-based meditation is focusing on a single word, such as "calm," "relax," "one," or "peace." The Beatles practiced a word (mantra)-focused Transcendental Meditation popularized by Maharishi Mahesh Yogi.

The most famous medical proponent of concentration meditation is Herbert Benson, M.D., the Harvard cardiologist and author of *The Relaxation Response* who founded the Benson-Henry Institute for Mind Body Medicine at the Massachusetts General Hospital. Over 35 years, Dr. Benson and his colleagues have documented the profound physical, mental, and emotional benefits of simple meditation practices, such as repeating the number "one." Concentration meditation builds attention, concentration, and confidence, as well as a sense of calm and peacefulness. It is similar to breathing meditation, but instead of counting breaths, simply repeat the number "one" or another word or phrase. When the mind wanders, gently bring it back to your chosen word.

To enhance the benefits, you can focus on a positive emotion, such as appreciation. You could also focus on a positive expectation or affirmation of hope—"I'm getting better; I can feel myself healing; help is on the way; yes, we can." You can also focus on a prayer or a short phrase of scripture to enhance the spiritual benefits of meditation.

Long-term meditation practice actually changes brain structure and function—it increases activity in the left-sided anterior prefrontal cortex (a pattern associated with positive moods) and the putamen (a part of the brain involved in attention and learning). Just as body builders develop larger muscles with practice, long-term meditators develop thicker, more active areas in the parts of the brain devoted to attention, processing, planning, and positive moods. Regular meditation practice leads to improved ability to cope, reduced pain, reduced anxiety, and enhanced immune function.

Here are three simple steps for concentration meditation.

Concentration Meditation

   1. Find a place where you will not be disturbed for the period

of your meditation; sit comfortably upright or recline with your spine straight so you feel supported and stable; set a timer so you don't have to look at a clock.

2. Pick a single object, word, phrase, emotion, or action on which to focus. Breathe in a relaxed, normal fashion. You don't have to take especially deep breaths, but you may notice your breathing gradually slows as you practice.

3. When your mind wanders, recognize it, refrain from self-criticism, and gently return your attention to your intended focus.

You may imagine your mind like an enthusiastic puppy you are taking for a walk. The puppy sees a squirrel (a sensation, thought, memory, plan, fantasy, or emotion) and darts toward it. You gently remind it to "heel." It does for a minute, and then it spots a leaf (another distracting thought or sensation) and darts toward that. You again remind it to "heel." Soon, it hears another dog (another distraction, like wondering if this is a waste of time and how much longer we have to do this), and it dashes to find a new friend. Again, "heel." Soon, the puppy mind, or as some call it, "monkey mind," learns to attend to the chosen object of attention, and concentration becomes effortless.

Mindfulness or Insight Meditation

Mindfulness meditation is a way of bringing your attention to the present moment, freeing your mind from ruminating about the past, judging anything, or worrying about the future. In mindfulness meditation, one is simply quietly aware of what is happening in the body, emotions, or thoughts, with kind curiosity, without judging those experiences, simply noticing how quickly the mind darts from physical sensation to emotion to thoughts, back to an emotion, on to thoughts of the past or future. As you notice a deviation from the present, simply notice it and return to awareness of the constantly changing present moment.

Mindfulness meditation is about being fully engaged in the present. The best-known scientific proponent of this form of meditation is Jon Kabat-Zinn, Ph.D., who founded the Center for Mindfulness in Medicine, Health Care, and Society at the University of Massachusetts. Dr. Kabat-Zinn and his colleagues globally have conducted numerous studies showing that mindfulness meditation improves anxiety, attention, mood, sleep, and stress[102].

Three Keys to Mindfulness Practice

There are three keys to mindfulness practice: intention, attitude, and attention.

1. *Intention:* Have a clear intention to focus on the present moment.

2. *Attitude:* Maintain a sense of curiosity and an open,

---

102 Kabat-Zinn J., et al., "Effectiveness of a meditation-based stress reduction program in the treatment of anxiety disorders," *Am J Psychiatry* 149, no. 7 (1992): 936–43. Zylowska, L., et al., "Mindfulness meditation training in adults and adolescents with ADHD: a feasibility study," *J Atten Disord* 11, no. 6 (2008): 737–46. Rosenzweig S., et al., "Mindfulness-based stress reduction lowers psychological distress in medical students," *Teach Learn Med* 15, no. 2 (2003): 88–92. Tang Y.Y., et al., "Short-term meditation training improves attention and self-regulation," *Proc Natl Acad Sci USA* 104, no. 43 (2007): 17152–6. Evans S., et al., "Mindfulness-based cognitive therapy for generalized anxiety disorder, *J Anxiety Disord* 22, no. 4 (2008): 716–21. Koszycki D., et al., "Randomized trial of a meditation-based stress reduction program and cognitive behavior therapy in generalized social anxiety disorder," *Behav Res Ther* 45, no. 10 (2007): 2518–26. Jain S., et al., "A randomized controlled trial of mindfulness meditation versus relaxation training: effects on distress, positive states of mind, rumination, and distraction," *Ann Behav Med* 33, no. 1 (2007): 11–21. Sephton S.E., et al., "Mindfulness meditation alleviates depressive symptoms in women with fibromyalgia: results of a randomized clinical trial," *Arthritis Rheum* 57, no. 1 (2007): 77–85. Winbush N.Y., et al., "The effects of mindfulness-based stress reduction on sleep disturbance: a systematic review," *Explore (NY)* 3, no. 6 (2007): 585–91.

accepting attitude about whatever emerges in one's perceptions, sensations, thoughts, or emotions during practice.

3. *Attention:* Focus on the present experience; when attention wanders to another time or place, return to present awareness, gently and without self-condemnation.

Three Ways to Start Practicing Mindfulness Meditation

There are three easy ways to practice mindfulness: body scan, sitting meditation, and moving meditation.

1. *Body scan:* For this practice, start with focusing on one tiny part of your body, such as your little toe. Be aware of any physical sensations in your little toe. Now move to the other toes, the rest of the foot, and so on up to the top of your head. Take your time. Just notice the sensations. You don't need to label them or judge whether they are good or bad. The focus is on awareness. You may notice that sensations change in unexpected ways. If you start thinking about something else, simply return your awareness to where you left off and begin again. Experienced meditators can take forty-five to sixty minutes to complete a body scan. Take your time. Do not worry if you take longer or shorter time than others. The OSU Center for Integrative Health and Wellness offers free guided practices for the body scan that you can download to your smart device from http://go.osu.edu/mindfulness. Similar recordings are available from the University of Wisconsin and the University of California at Los Angeles.

2. *Sitting meditation:* For this meditation, sit in a comfortable position. Become aware of your breathing, the sounds in the

room, the quality of light, aromas, and other perceptions. Imagine that you are a three-month-old baby who does not yet have names for things, so you can just observe without labeling or judging. When a thought other than your current perception enters your mind, notice it, and return to observing and perceiving the current moment. Similarly, emotions need not be rejected or avoided; just note the emotions that arise. Neither pursue nor flee them. Simply observe in a curious, neutral, detached way. When judgments or criticisms arise, similarly notice them and set them aside. Soon you will notice how quickly thoughts and judgments come and go. What remains is the awareness of awareness.

3. *Movement:* Dr. Kabat-Zinn, the Kripalu Center for Yoga & Health, and others include gentle hatha yoga and walking meditation as a type of mindfulness meditation practice. Others might include tai chi or QiGong exercises. These kinds of exercises are typically done very slowly and gently and can be readily adapted or modified if discomfort is encountered. Slow, conscious movement that is not aimed specifically at achieving any goal other than awareness of the movement itself can provide the same benefits as sitting and body scan meditations. That is, it can improve memory, attention, concentration, and mood, while decreasing worry and obsessive thoughts[103].

Mindfulness can be incorporated into any other kind of exercise, whether it is weightlifting, swimming, or running. It can also be

---

103 Chattha R., et al., "Effect of yoga on cognitive functions in climacteric syndrome: a randomised control study," *BJOG* 115, no. 8 (2008): 991–1000.

included in other daily activities—eating, washing dishes, brushing teeth, participating in conversations, gardening, creating art or music, answering the phone. Eventually, you may want to bring mindful awareness to every moment of your life.

Concentration and meditation practices are just two types of mind-body skills. Another useful set of skills involves imagery and visualization. We started to explore the use of visualization and harnessing the power of imagination in Chapter 6. Additional exercises are described below. Wise healers become familiar with a variety of tools to use for themselves and their patients. Gaining experience with a range of practices will help you select those that are most helpful for you in different situations. Not everyone is a visual person. Even if you don't visualize easily, you may want to review the following exercises—you never know when they might come in handy.

Guided Imagery, Visualization

Let's review five different examples of guided imagery or visualization practices:

1. Visualizing a natural object or setting that engenders a sense of serenity and safety
2. Nature's peace
3. Seeking counsel from a wise guide
4. Being part of a circle of caring healers
5. Visualizing healing colors.

You can practice guided imagery or visualization on your own, with a CD or DVD, a YouTube video, or with professional guidance.

For any of the exercises here, feel free to read the directions to make a recording of your own voice talking you through the imagery to guide you as you practice. Safe, serene place, wise guide, and caring circle images are widely used by health professionals who offer guided imagery, including Dr. James Gordon at the Center for Mind-Body Medicine. Belleruth Naparstek at HealthJourneys.com offers a diverse array of guided imagery recordings.

Practice regularly to develop your skills and deepen your sense of well-being.

1. Imagery for a Serene, Safe Place

- Sit or lay in a comfortable position. Focus on your breathing. Relax your belly. Allow your arms and legs to relax and feel warm and comfortable. You may want to start with a few minutes of Progressive Muscle Relaxation or Autogenic Training to start the relaxation process.
- Imagine yourself in a place where you feel *safe* and *content*. It might be a place in nature, such as the beach, a waterfall, the woods, or a mountain. It might be a particular tree or rock. It could be indoors in your favorite room. It could be a real place or a place from a movie, a book, or your imagination. It's your experience; you get to choose.
- Engage your senses. How does this place look? What do you see? Is it bright or dim? What colors are dominant? What do you hear? Is it quiet? Are there natural sounds? Favorite music? Pleasant aromas? Have you just eaten? Are you about to eat? Have you just awakened from a restful sleep? Done some vigorous exercise? Ready to run? Are you drowsy and about to nap? Is there someone with you—a person, a pet, an

animal, a plant, an imaginary being? Feel free to add things or rearrange them until they are just the way you like.

- Imagine yourself in this place feeling safe, secure, and serene, calm, content, relaxed, focused, and confident; dwell on the images; notice how your body feels.
- Rest in this safe, serene place as long as you like and return as often as you like.

If you have trouble remembering such a place, use your imagination to create a vivid scene of your own special secure, enjoyable place. The brain responds to imaginary images as if they were actually occurring, sending signals to your entire body that improve mood, sleep, and immune function while decreasing anxiety and stress. Sometimes it is enough to simply be in a place where you feel safe and comfortable to allow your intuition to guide you. Sometimes it is helpful to engage your imagination to seek additional help from deep within. This is a good time to ask for guidance from your inner wise guide.

2. Nature's Peace

One of my favorite imagery practices was taught by Dora Kunz, one of the founders of Therapeutic Touch. She began many of our practice sessions together with this imagery.

- Sit or lay in a comfortable position with your spine straight.
- Imagine yourself in a beautiful, safe place in nature. It might be the beach or the mountains, a meadow, a stream, or a peaceful lake. You may decide to focus on a large, stable rock formation or a single tree.

- As you gaze at this part of Nature, feel its deep peace. Breathe this peace into your heart.
- Now say to yourself, "I am that peace." Affirm that with each breath: "I am that peace."
- Feel that you are a part of Nature, that you and Nature are radiating this peace out into the world.
- Rest in that sense of peace and connection for several minutes, then gradually stretch and return to ordinary awareness.

You can download a free MP3 recording of this practice from the Ohio State University Center for Integrative Health and Wellness website: http://go.osu.edu/heartpractices.

3. Imagery for a Wise Guide

There are times we each seek wise guidance. An older relative, a trusted friend, a teacher, or mentor can offer guidance or supportive listening. Even when such a person is not physically available, there is a source of wisdom within you that you can tap with your imagination. Here's how:

- Sit or lay in a comfortable position. Focus on your breathing. Relax your belly. Allow your arms and legs to relax and feel warm and comfortable.
- Imagine yourself in your safe place. You may want to practice Autogenic Training or Progressive Muscle Relaxation for a few minutes to become more deeply relaxed. Then visit your safe, serene place to deepen that sense of relaxation.
- Ask your inner wise guide to join you here for a little while.

- Notice the first person, animal, or imaginary creature that enters your safe space. It may be a real person from your current life or your past, a wise historical figure, a poet, a philosopher, or a healer. It could be an animal or a bird; it could be a fantasy figure or a character from mythology or cartoons.
- Welcome this being and thank it for joining you. Tell your guide your intention.
- Ask your question.
- Listen. Don't worry if you don't hear right away. Sometimes the answer comes in her expression or the way the wise guide sits or stands or something she hands you or some other action. Sometimes you will realize what the answer is after you've finished the exercise.
- Thank the wise guide for coming and sharing her wisdom. Tell her how you will honor and use this advice to achieve your highest intention.
- Return to an awareness of your breathing and your body; notice how you feel now. Jot down any impressions or ideas in your journal.

Sometimes we yearn simply for a sense of being surrounded by caring and compassionate beings that have our best interests at heart. This is a good time to practice the guided imagery of the caring circle.

4. Imagery for a Caring Circle

- Sit or lay in a comfortable position. Focus on your breathing. Relax your belly. Allow your arms and legs to relax and feel warm and comfortable. You may want to do a few minutes of

Autogenic Training practice or Progressive Muscle Relaxation to deepen your relaxation.

- Imagine yourself in your safe, serene place. Remind yourself of your intention.
- Notice that this place is large enough for others to join you. As you sit, you notice that there are chairs or cushions arranged all around you. Soon, others come to sit in these chairs. Each place is filled with someone who shares your intention to serve to help others and who holds your best interest at heart; someone who wants you to experience happiness, confidence, success, and joy; someone who is proud of you and knows you are a good person deep down. Each one may be someone you know—a relative, friend, or teacher. They could be historical, cartoon, or mythical figures who showed great compassion, love, kindness, or healing ability during their lifetime and who now come to share that caring and compassion with you. They are all joined in wanting the best for you. You may not have understood before how deeply they are connected to one another, to Nature, and to you, but now you can feel that connection.
- Feel their love and appreciation for you; feel yourself growing stronger and yet softer, more capable, and more kind. Notice how you feel sitting in the middle of this circle of caring and compassionate beings.
- Sit and receive their care and compassion. As you breathe in, take in deep breaths of their powerful healing presence. As you breathe out, extend your gratitude and compassion to them. Repeat this for several minutes.
- Silently thank them for coming and sharing their love, wisdom, and inspiration with you.

- Return to an awareness of your breathing and your body; notice how you feel now. Jot down any impressions or ideas in your journal.

With guided imagery, you may modify the images to suit your goals. You can repeat the practices as often as you like.

5. Visualization with Colors

Many healers visualize colors while healing. You can encourage the recipient to collaborate and participate in the healing process by visualizing colors, too. The colors most often used in healing work are royal blue (to promote a sense of calm, peace, and comfort), green (to promote a sense of balance and dynamic equilibrium), and white or golden yellow (to empower, detoxify, energize, or promote vitality)[104].

Healing Colors

Red, orange, and peach are very rarely used in healing. They may be excessively stimulating. I have used red on some occasions to "run" energy into the feet of patients suffering from fatigue, but this can lead to a sense of uncomfortable agitation. In general, it is better to visualize a calm, orderly golden yellow to promote a sense of vitality. The rose-pink color can be helpful to someone who is grieving or frightened.

Colors can mean different things to different people. The listing of qualities associated with colors in this table is a general guide, not the absolute, invariant truth for every individual.

104 Krieger D., *Accepting Your Power to Heal: the Personal Practice of Therapeutic Touch*, (Santa Fe: Bear and Company, 1993), 180.

Colors	Qualities
Clear	Clarity, openness, permeability
Gold/yellow	Vitality, moving, invigorating, stimulating, warm, nurturing
Green	Balance, equilibrium, dynamic stability, organized, harmony
Purple or violet	Devotion, dedication, blessing, sacred, aspirational
Rose/pink	Love, affection, acceptance, gentleness, sympathy, safety, trust, optimism
Royal blue	Comfortable, tranquil, orderly, coherent, quiet, cool, serene, graceful
White	Detoxifying, purifying, empowering

Keep a Journal

In the chapter on Emotional Preparation, we discussed keeping a gratitude journal as one way of promoting an attitude of gratitude. Journals can be helpful in other ways, too.

Writing down experiences is a good way to understand them better and to understand ourselves and our deepest values, wants, and needs. Scientific research supports the benefits of keeping a journal on promoting a sense of well-being, improving sleep, and decreasing stress, anxiety, and depression[105].

---

105 Chung, C.K. and J.W. Pennebaker, "Variations in the spacing of expressive writing sessions," Br J Health Psychol 13 Pt. 1 (2008): 15–21. Swanbon T., et al., "Expressive writing reduces avoidance and somatic complaints in a community sample with constraints on expression, Br J Health Psychol 13 Pt. 1 (2008): 53–6. Smyth J.M., et al., "Expressive writing and post-traumatic stress disorder: effects on trauma symptoms, mood states, and cortisol reactivity," Br J Health Psychol 13 Pt. 1 (2008): 85–93. Gortner E.M., et al., "Benefits of expressive writing in lowering rumination and depressive symptoms," Behav Ther 37, no. 3 (2006): 292–303.

What are the downsides of keeping a journal? As with any new practice, it takes time you used to spend on something else. A few people notice that things seem to get worse shortly after they start, whereas others have a temporary sense of complete resolution, and still others notice nothing different; all of these can be misleading. While it's sometimes true that things get worse before they get better or people experience miraculous healing, it's best to stick with a practice for at least three to six weeks to get a realistic sense of its effects on you.

What are the benefits? Besides improving yourself awareness, mood, and sleep, you can also use a journal to document your dreams, your ideas, your different practices, and your healing experiences. This will help you identify patterns you may not have noticed before and lead to greater insight and wisdom[106]. In particular, tracking your healing sessions is very useful.

Tips for Keeping a Journal

- Keep it simple.
- Find a notebook, software program, or recording device that suits you.
- Make it convenient and easy so you will use it frequently.
- Note the date and time of each entry. You may want to add a couple of keywords or events to the top of the entry so you can find it easily again when you want to review.
- Note what you observe, think, dream, wonder, eat, drink, feel, or experience. Write whatever seems relevant to you.

---

106 Lyubomirsky S.L., et al., "The costs and benefits of writing, talking, and thinking about life's triumphs and defeats," *J Pers Soc Psychol* 90, no. 4 (2006): 692–708.

Do not worry about grammar, spelling, or punctuation. You do not need to share the contents with anyone else. If you feel like drawing a picture or doodling instead, do that.

Let's look at one more mental preparation practice before we move to the next chapter.

Biofeedback

Biofeedback is a modern technology that provides moment-to-moment information about some aspect of your own physiologic state. Remember mood rings? When you felt stressed, they turned yellow, red, or black, and when you were relaxed and happy, they turned dark blue. Mood rings are very simple thermal (temperature) biofeedback devices. They work on the principle that when we're stressed, the blood vessels in our fingers contract (so more blood goes to the large muscles enabling us to fight or flee), making our fingers cooler; when we're more relaxed, the blood vessels in our fingers relax, more blood flows, and they are warmer.

For the past fifteen years, I have enjoyed practicing biofeedback as a way of helping me focus during meditation, and to help remind me when my mind has wandered. I also love gadgets and devices, and I love being able to track my physiologic changes with practice. Time and again, I've noticed subtle physiologic changes with my biofeedback-augmented practice before I noticed any symptoms. This early warning system helps me take steps early to prevent deterioration and promote vitality.

An increasing number of systems are available for home computers and smart devices. The two that I've used most are Healing Rhythms™ from Wild Divine and emWave™ from the Institute of

HeartMath. These systems allow you to connect a small device from your finger or earlobe to the computer or smartphone or tablet. The device gathers information about your heart rate, skin temperature, or skin moisture. The computer transforms the information from your body into images, sounds, or games that allow you to learn to regulate your own physiology. Another system, RespErate™, has approval from the FDA as a way of lowering blood pressure.

You don't need to buy a biofeedback device to learn to meditate or use guided imagery. These devices can be fun ways to augment your preparation for healing, but they are not necessary. We sometimes use them in workshops to demonstrate how powerfully our mental images and mental states affect our physiology.

Summary Table for Mental Preparation Practices for Healing

We've covered physical, emotional, and mental preparation. There's just one more category of preparation before we dive into the healing practices themselves: spiritual preparation. Don't worry; spiritual preparation does not require any kind of religious belief. Curious? That's what the next chapter is all about.

Practice	Purpose/Description
Concentration-type Meditation	Build attention skills. Focus on a single word or other object; when attention wanders, notice that and return attention to the chosen word or object.
Mindfulness-type or Insight Meditation	Build present-centered, non-judgmental awareness and insight. Set an intention to be aware of the present moment; maintain a sense of curiosity and friendliness; when attention wanders, bring it back to the present. Body scan Seated meditation Yoga, walking, or other gentle moving meditation
Guided Imagery/Visualization	Achieve a specific goal using imagination. Typically start with brief Autogenic Training or Progressive Muscle Relaxation to relax fully before engaging imagination: Safe, serene place Nature's peace Counsel from a wise guide Becoming part of a caring circle of colleagues Visualizing colors with specific healing qualities
Journaling	Increased self-awareness and pattern recognition.
Biofeedback	Increased sense of self-control and self-confidence. Recognition that mental and emotional states profoundly affect physiology. Healing Rhythms™ HeartMath EmWave PSR™ or Inner Balance™ app

CHAPTER 9

Spiritual Practices to Prepare for Healing Work

*"At the deepest level, the creative process and the healing
process arise from a single source. When you are an artist,
you are a healer; a wordless trust of the same mystery is
the foundation of your work and its integrity."*

—RACHEL NAOMI REMEN, M.D.

YOU DON'T HAVE TO BE RELIGIOUS or believe in a particular deity and you
don't have to be a professional artist or musician to engage in spiritual practices to prepare for healing work. Spiritual practices relate to
a sense of meaning and purpose (Chapter 1) and to something greater
than our individual selves. This could be the sacred, to a higher power, principle, or presence; or it could be the long lineage of healers
worldwide who have dedicated themselves to the relief of suffering;
it could be Nature, music, or art. Spiritual practices help us transcend
our individual notion of our separate selves. The spiritual practices
discussed here include:

- Prayer
- Ritual
- Storytelling and literature

- Dreams
- Art, creative expression
- Music
- Nature

Prayer

Prayer is a very ancient practice, part of every indigenous culture, a way to connect with the sacred or divine power, or a principle or spirit greater than our individual selves. Prayer may also be defined as a deeply and reverently held intention directed toward a higher power or God. There are many kinds of prayer: prayers of gratitude and thanksgiving, of praise, for understanding, for healing, for direction, for sustenance, for faith, for ourselves, and for others. The writer Anne Lamott summarized all prayers into three words: "help," "thanks," and "wow."[107] These simple words succinctly capture the healer's heartfelt intention to relieve suffering (help), gratitude for the ability to serve that calling (thanks), and awe in the presence of the mystery of healing (wow). Regardless of the type of prayer, regular practice of a deeply held intention helps focus the mind and may be considered a type of focused attention meditation.

Numerous scientific studies show that, in general, people who pray regularly enjoy better health than those who do not[108]. For example, prayer can reduce stress, ease anxiety, diminish depression,

---

107 Lamott A., *Help, Thanks, Wow: The Three Essential Prayers*, (New York: Riverhead Hardcover, 2012).
108 Levin J., "Spiritual determinants of health and healing: an epidemiologic perspective on salutogenic mechanisms," *Altern Ther Health Med* 9, no. 6 (2003): 48–57. Bormann J.E.,et al., "Efficacy of frequent mantram repetition on stress, quality of life, and spiritual well-being in veterans: a pilot study," *J Holist Nurs* 23, no. 4 (2005): 395–414. Bormann J.E., et al., "Effects of spiritual mantram repetition on HIV outcomes: a randomized controlled trial," *J Behav Med* 29, no. 4 (2006): 359–76.

and substantially lower the risk of suicide[109]. In a study of health care professionals who were trained to frequently repeat a word with spiritual significance (a form of prayer or spiritual practice), there were significant improvements in stress, anxiety, and well-being[110]. Furthermore, some people who *expect* to receive prayer from others enjoy a greater sense of well-being than those who do not[111]. On the other hand, a 2009 analysis of ten studies evaluating the effectiveness of intercessory prayer as a complementary therapy for people with health problems concluded that there was no significant effect on death, re-hospitalization, or re-admission to the coronary care unit[112]. Expectation of the benefits of prayer may raise hopes and offer comfort, but one study actually showed that some patients who were certain they were receiving prayer had more complications than patients who were not certain about receiving prayer[113].

In short, the scientific data on praying for others are mixed in terms of its effects on measurable health outcomes. However, the scientific data clearly show that those who engage in prayer enjoy better physical, mental, and emotional health. Therefore, if consistent with personal beliefs, prayer is a reasonable practice for healers to engage in for their own well-being and to prepare to serve others. Healers typically pray to develop a stronger recognition of their

---

109 Larson D.B., "Religion and Mental Health: Should they work together?" *Alternative & Complementary Therapies*, (Mar/April 1996): 91–98.
110 Bormann J.E., et al., "Relationship of frequent mantram repetition to emotional and spiritual well-being in healthcare workers," *J Contin Educ Nurs* 37, no. 5 (2006): 218–24.
111 Meisenhelder J.B., et al., "Prayer and health outcomes in church members," *Altern Ther Health Med* 6, no. 4 (2000): 56–60.
112 Roberts L., et al., "Intercessory prayer for the alleviation of ill health," *Cochrane Database Syst Rev*, (April 15, 2009): CD000368.
113 Benson H., et al., "Study of the Therapeutic Effects of Intercessory Prayer (STEP) in cardiac bypass patients: a multicenter randomized trial of uncertainty and certainty in receiving intercessory prayer," *Am Heart J* 151, no. 4 (2006): 934–42.

connection with God, Spirit, or Universal healing energy, the source of healing—in themselves and in those for whom they pray.

Prayer can include recitation of memorized prayers, scripture, hymns, mantras, or sacred texts (such as the famous Serenity Prayer recited in many AA meetings):

"God grant us the serenity to accept the things we cannot change,
courage to change the things we can,
and wisdom to know the difference."

—Reinhold Niebuhr

Ritual Practices to Promote Centering and Grounding

Professional health care practices are filled with modern rituals, such as reciting the Hippocratic Oath at medical school graduations and wearing white coats or uniforms in hospitals and clinics. Rituals help create a sense of identity and connection with the larger group or tradition of healing.

In many indigenous healing practices, a healing session begins by introducing all of those present, stating the reason for the session, and calling on the powers of the four directions (east, south, west, and north), as well as the power of the earth and sky, to assist in the healing process. Some traditions also call on the four (or five) elements: earth, air, water, fire, and space (or life). It is also common to call upon the wisdom of the ancestors of the patient and the healer to bring collective wisdom and power to bear on the work at hand. Many shamans follow an invocation of the powers of the directions and/or elements by calling on the power of plants, creatures that live in the sea and sky, and animals of the earth, and follow this invocation with rhythmic drumming or chanting. To the extent that these practices are consistent with your beliefs, values, and culture, they can assist in strengthening the sense of being centered and grounded.

Reflect on what kinds of ritual are most meaningful for you and those with whom you work. The type of ritual may vary depending on the setting. While you may light a candle at home, open flames are contra-indicated in most hospitals. No matter how "cool" or exotic a practice is, if it feels inauthentic to you, do not use it in your healing work. It is important that your preparatory practices contribute to, rather than distract from, being centered and grounded in the practical work of caring. If a practice makes you or the recipient uncomfortable, avoid it.

Storytelling and Literature

It's often inspiring and uplifting to see, hear, or read about others who have met similar challenges. Healers may wish to read stories or great literature about other healers and about patients who recovered from difficult illnesses.

It can also be therapeutic for healers to listen to the stories of those who come for help. This is called "narrative medicine." Serving as a supportive person who will be present along the journey with one who is suffering is a form of empathy and social support, which in itself is therapeutic. Narratives often embody the meaning of the illness or provide clues to its cause or cure. They can help foster reflection and a sense of common humanity to understand the person who is suffering, as well as the disease or injury afflicting him.

Dreams

The great psychologist, Carl Jung, posited that dreams connected the dreamer with the collective unconscious. Thus, dreams connect us not only to our own unconscious physiologic processes, but also to one another. In this way, paying attention to our dreams is a spiritual activity because dreams connect us to something greater than our individual, conscious sense of self.

When I was a pediatrician-in-training, my tasks included doing a daily physical examination for each child under my care in the hospital. This was usually done first thing in the morning, and the children were often groggy and grumpy. Not only were they sick, but I was waking them up, not for breakfast, but a physical exam. One morning I walked into a very sick girl's room and was greeted by her wide-awake enthusiasm. I was surprised because she had recently received a bone marrow transplant, which is usually associated with fatigue and a high rate of infections because the immune system is suppressed and the white blood cell count is low. "You seem really happy this morning," I noted. "What's happened?" She did not hesitate, "My white count is going to be up today!" I wondered what would make her think so since her blood test was not scheduled until later that morning, and yesterday's count had been in the cellar. "I had a dream that I watched a thermometer. I saw the mercury go up, up, up, and that means my white count is going up!" she explained with glee. Sure enough, several hours later, her test showed that her white blood cell count had indeed gone up, up, up.

That girl's story has stayed with me for over thirty years and has inspired me to ask many more patients about their dreams. While modern science doesn't have a clear explanation about how we generate the content of our dreams, it is clear that they can provide a window into unconscious physiologic processes. Dreams have warned about impending bladder infections, pneumonia, and fevers, as well as recoveries. Dreams have suggested treatments and remedies for me and for my patients. In many cultures, one of a healer's most important jobs is to listen to and interpret dreams for members of the community.

Creative or Artistic Expression

Numerous studies have shown the mental and physical health benefits of engaging in artistic expression[114]. Some healing traditions explicitly draw on practices, such as sand painting or creating mandalas, as part of the healing process.

Art is a way of expressing ourselves and connecting us to larger ideas or images. Being fully engaged in activities that are absorbing or challenging, such as creating art, music, literature, or poetry, shifts our attention to this moment and enhances a sense of well-being and connection to something meaningful. Being fully engaged in an activity in which the challenge level is high and one's skills are fully used to meet that challenge results in what one of my college professors, Mihaly Csikszentmihalyi, Ph.D., calls *flow*. This state is commonly experienced during intense absorption in creative

---

114 Pratt R.R., "Art, dance, and music therapy," *Phys Med Rehabil Clin N Am* 15, no. 4 (2004): 827–41. Hannemann B.T., "Creativity with dementia patients. Can creativity and art stimulate dementia patients positively?," *Gerontology* 52, no. 1 (2006): 59–65. Garland S.N., et al., "A non-randomized comparison of mindfulness-based stress reduction and healing arts programs for facilitating post-traumatic growth and spirituality in cancer outpatients," *Support Care Cancer* 15, no. 8 (2007): 949–61. Hamre H.J., et al., "Anthroposophic therapy for chronic depression: a four-year prospective cohort study," *BMC Psychiatry* 6 (2006): 57.

endeavors[115]. The quality of absorption is much more important than the quality of the outcome product in terms of promoting the ability to remain centered. You don't need to wait for a professional to get started with (or get back to) creative work that brings you a sense of happiness or contentment that nurtures your healing work.

By engaging in the arts, music, dance, and creative expression, people can actively mourn, grieve, celebrate, find inner power to endure their situation, and find healing and meaning. An analysis of over a dozen studies of art therapy for patients with breast cancer showed that even under that trying circumstance, engaging in art therapy effectively lowered anxiety[116]. Art can be particularly helpful in expressing, understanding, and healing emotions and thoughts, especially for people who have difficulty finding words to express themselves.

Music

Music's beneficial health effects have been known for thousands of years. Ancient philosophers from Plato to Confucius and the kings of Israel sang the praises of music and used it to help soothe stress. Military bands use music to build confidence and courage. Sporting events provide music to rouse enthusiasm. Schoolchildren use music to memorize their ABCs. Shopping malls play music to entice consumers and keep them in the store. Dentists play music to help calm nervous patients; others use music to beat the blues[117].

---

115 Csikszentmihalyi M., *Creativity: Flow and the Psychology of Discovery and Invention*, (New York: Harper Perennial, 1997).
116 Boehm K., et al., "Arts therapies for anxiety, depression, and quality of life in breast cancer patients: a systematic review and meta-analysis," *Evid Based Complement Altern Med*, (Feb 16, 2014): 103297.
117 Maratos A, et al., "Music therapy for depression," *Cochrane Database Syst Rev* 1 (2008): CD004517. Kamioka H., et al., "Effectiveness of music therapy: a summary of systematic reviews based on randomized controlled trials of music interventions," *Patient Prefer Adherence*, (May 16 2014): 727–54.

Modern research supports conventional wisdom that music benefits health. Different kinds of music have different effects. Some kinds rouse soldiers to battle, while others can decrease aggression and improve sociability[118], and yet others are used to ease into sleep[119]. It is important for healers to be aware of the effects music has on them and the different kinds of people they serve—the kind of music that is soothing to a three-year-old may be irritating to a teenager and have minimal effects on an adult.

Because of our unique experiences, we develop different musical tastes and preferences. Despite these differences, there are some common, scientifically established responses to music. Certain kinds of music make almost everyone feel worse, even when someone says she enjoys it; in a study of 144 adults and teenagers who listened to four different kinds of music, grunge music led to significant increases in hostility, sadness, tension, and fatigue across the entire group, even in the teenagers who said they liked it[120]. In another study, college students reported that pop, rock, oldies, and classical music helped them feel happier and more optimistic, friendly, relaxed, and calm[121].

Binaural Beats

Any kind of relaxing, calming, slow-to-moderate tempo music in major keys can contribute to calmer moods. Some studies suggest

118 Rickson, D.J. and W.G. Watkins, "Music therapy to promote prosocial behaviors in aggressive adolescent boys—a pilot study," *J Music Ther* 40, no. 4 (2003): 283–301.
119 Lai H.L., et al., "Music improves sleep quality in older adults," *J Adv Nurs* 49, no. 3 (2005): 234–44. Hernandez-Ruiz, E., "Effect of music therapy on the anxiety levels and sleep patterns of abused women in shelters," *J Music Ther* 42, no. 2 (2005): 140–58. Harmat L., et al., "Music improves sleep quality in students," *J Adv Nurs* 62, no. 3 (2008): 327–35.
120 McCraty R., et al., "The effects of different types of music on mood, tension, and mental clarity," *Altern Ther Health Med* 4, no. 1 (1998): 75–84.
121 Stratton V.N., "Influence of music and socializing on perceived stress while waiting," *Percept Mot Skills* 75, no. 1 (1992): 334.

that specially designed music, such as music that includes tones that intentionally induce *binaural beats* to put brain waves into relaxed delta or theta rhythms, can help improve anxiety even more than music without these tones[122]. Healers interested in experiencing the effects of binaural beats on their own mental and emotional state should listen to this music with headphones and not while driving, cooking, operating dangerous equipment, or supervising small children. It may make you drowsy, particularly if you listen to binaural beats that induce alpha, theta, or delta brainwaves. The good news about drowsiness-inducing music is that it can help promote better sleep[123].

Sounds from Nature

Many people find sounds from nature, such as oceans, streams, rain, birdsong, and similar sounds, to be very soothing and comforting. Sounds from everyday life, such as morning birdsong and evening cricket chirps, can help us feel more connected to the rhythm of daily life and keep us oriented to day-night cycles that are sometimes obscured in environments with constant exposure to bright light.

---

122 Padmanabhan R., et al., "A prospective, randomized, controlled study examining binaural beat audio and pre-operative anxiety in patients undergoing general anesthesia for day case surgery," *Anesthesia* 60, no. 9 (2005): 874–7. Le Scouarnec R.P., et al., "Use of binaural beat tapes for treatment of anxiety: a pilot study of tape preference and outcomes," *Altern Ther Health Med* 7, no. 1 (2001): 58–63. Wahbeh H., et al., "Binaural beat technology in humans: a pilot study to assess psychologic and physiologic effects," *J Altern Complement Med* 13, no.1 (2007): 25–32. Weiland T.J., et al., "Original sound compositions reduce anxiety in emergency department patients: a randomized controlled trial," *Med J Aust*, 2011; 195 (11–12): 694–8.
123 Abeln V., et al., "Brainwave entrainment for better sleep and post-sleep state of young elite soccer players—a pilot study," *Eur J Sport Sci* 14, no. 15 (2014): 393–402.

Nature

Spending time in nature can be both a spiritual and a healing experience. Being in the midst of a forest, meadow, on a mountain or near a stream, lake, or ocean helps use recognize our place in the natural world.

One of my favorite places is the Grand Canyon. No matter how many pictures or movies I'd seen, when I first saw the Grand Canyon in person, I was awestruck. It is so enormous that it takes your breath away. Sitting near the edge of the Grand Canyon, I felt in my bones how small my life was compared to the vastness of geologic time. Seeing the stars at night made me realize that as vast as the Grand Canyon is, our planet is just one among many planets in a giant Universe. This experience was both calming and uplifting, humbling and energizing. That's the power of Nature!

Exposure to a natural environment, to gardens and parks, helps improve health[124]. It can reduce mental fatigue[125]. It can promote more focused attention. In Japan, the practice of intentionally spending time in nature for health has a name: forest therapy[126]. Even looking through a window at a natural environment helps promote

---

124 Song C., et al., "Physiological and psychological effects of walking on young males in urban parks in winter," *J Physiol Anthropol*, 2013;Oct 29; 32: 18.
125 Tanaka M, et al., "Fatigue-recovering effect of a house designed with open space," *Explore* 9, no. 2 (2013): 82–86.
126 Lee J., et al., "Influence of forest therapy on cardiovascular relaxation in young adults," *Evid Based Complement Alt Med*, (2014): 834360.

shorter hospital stays in surgical patients[127]. Likewise, the presence of ornamental plants in hospital rooms speeds surgical recovery[128]. Begun in 1978, the Planetree organization includes more than 500 organizations in eight countries working to help transform health care by providing empowering patient-centered care offered in a healing environment[129].

I encourage healers to spend time in nature regularly. Walk barefoot so your body is in direct contact with Mother Earth. Rest with your back against the tree and sense its vitality. Listen to the birds, contemplate the ocean, feel the wind in your face. Spending time in Nature helps us feel more grounded and more centered, renewed and refreshed for our healing work.

Summary of Spiritual Healing Preparation Practices

Before diving into warm-up exercises for healing, let's explore in more depth in Part 2 preparation for healing by becoming more familiar with modern and ancient healing. That's what Chapter 10 is all about.

127 Ulrich R.S. "View through a window may influence recovery from surgery," *Science* 224, no. 4647 (1984): 420–1.
128 Park S.H., et al., "Ornamental indoor plants in hospital rooms enhanced health outcomes of patients recovering from surgery," *J Altern Complement Med* 15, no. 9 (2009): 975–80.
129 Find out more about the Planetree model and organizations that have adopted it at http://planetree.org.

Practice	Purpose
Prayer	Strengthen connection with a higher power or greater presence. Affirm values. Improve personal health. Centering and grounding.
Ritual	Strengthen centering and grounding. Affirm connection with culture, tradition, community of healers, and values.
Storytelling, Narrative, and Literature	Strengthen empathy. Become inspired and hopeful. Gain insights into etiology and possible treatments.
Dreams	Connection with collective and personal unconscious. Develop insight and cues about causes and possible treatments.
Art and Creative or Artistic Expression	Connecting with collective and personal unconscious, meaning, purpose; creativity; connection with non-verbal insights and ideas.
Music	Calming, soothing, uplifting; connection with non-verbal ideas; assist with sleep and stress reduction.
Nature	Connecting with healing power of nature; promote focused, yet open attention.

CHAPTER 10

Modern and Ancient Anatomy for Healers

Modern Medicine and Anatomy

Long before *Grey's Anatomy* became a popular television program, it was the name of the textbook used in medical schools. Before we were allowed to touch a patient, we had to understand anatomy. Nurses, physical therapists, and many other healing professionals dedicate many hours to the study of anatomy. You don't have to be a health professional to benefit from understanding anatomy, and nowadays there are beautiful, inexpensive coloring books available to help you review the basics[130]. Before we dive into the ancient anatomy ideas that form the basis for several healing techniques, let's review the basics of the modern anatomy of flowing fluids and electromagnetic energies, starting with the heart.

---

130 Personally, I learned the most in anatomy from drawing and re-drawing the different parts I needed to learn. Drawing helps create a concrete connection from the hand to the brain. I encourage healers to find a book that resonates with them and draw images of all the anatomic structures described in this chapter.

1. Cardiovascular Anatomy

Everyone knows the heart pumps blood throughout the body. Did you know the heart actually has a pair of pumps (ventricles) and two holding tanks (atria)? The right side of the heart receives blood from the body, accumulates it in a holding tank "atrium," and then the right ventricle sends the "used" blood into the lungs to exchange carbon dioxide for fresh oxygen. The left side of the heart receives the freshly oxygenated blood from the lungs in the left atrium holding tank and pumps it out through the aorta and major vessels to the rest of the body. The cycle repeats second after second, minute after minute, whether you are awake or asleep, eating or walking, reading or driving. The body's wisdom monitors each organ's needs and adjusts accordingly. Marvelous!

The double-pump in our hearts is one of the strongest, steadiest innate rhythms we have. But what makes the heart pump? And how does it know how hard and how fast to go? There is a tiny collection of nerves, a mini-brain, in the right atrium of the heart that generates the electro-magnetic impulses that trigger the muscles that power the pumps. This mini-brain also sends signals to the head-brain, starting with a small collection of nerves (the cardio-pulmonary plexus) just above the heart that feeds information through a big nerve (the vagus) to let the brain know what's going on in the heart.

In turn, the brain signals the heart (back through the vagus nerve) to adjust the heart rate and pumping strength ("Something is scary and we may need to run, get ready to speed up and pump harder." "She's planning to sit down and eat, slow down and send more blood to the stomach."). The lungs and heart share a close connection of nerves through the cardio-pulmonary plexus so they can work harmoniously. Hormones circulating in the blood provide chemical signals about blood pressure, salt balance, stress, and other factors that influence the strength and speed of the pump. A complex orchestra of many instruments plays the heart's rhythmic music.

The heart's electromagnetic signal is so strong that its field can be measured all the way down in the ankles (with ECG, electrocardiogram, leads), and even several feet outside the body with a sensitive device called a SQUID (Super-Conducting Quantum Interference Device). Does that electromagnetic signal affect anything other than the heart?

Good question! The ECG's electro-magnetic signals are so strong that they are found in the brain waves, or EEG. People who study EEGs have to filter out the "noise" of the ECG in order to focus on the EEG. Drs. Linda Russek and Gary Schwartz at the University of Arizona have even found ECG signals from one person's heart in the EEG (brainwaves) of another person's brain[131]. This means that that pattern of your heart's electromagnetic signals can be found in a nearby person's brain waves. Even more surprising, studies by Dr. Rollin McCraty at the U.S. Institute of HeartMath have shown that the heart shows signs of intuition, responding to emotional stimuli with changes in the ECG slightly *before* they are presented to research subjects, and microseconds before the brain's EEG responds[132]. Does this mean the heart is more intuitive than the brain? More research is needed to better understand the answer to that question.

---

131 http://www.ssporer.com/downloads/Energetic_Heart.pdf. Russek L.G. and Schwartz G.E., "Interpersonal and heart-brain registration and the perception of parental love: a 42-year follow-up of the Harvard Mastery of Stress Study," *Subtle Energies* 5, no. 3 (1994): 195–208.
132 McCraty R., et al., "Electrophysiological evidence of intuition: part 1. The surprising role of the heart," *J Altern Complement Med* 10, no. 1 (2004): 133–43. McCraty R., et al., "Electrophysiological evidence of intuition: part 2. A system-wide process?," *J Altern Complement Med* 10, no. 2 (2004): 325–36.

2. The Lymphatic System

The lymphatic system is sometimes considered part of the cardiovascular system because one of its main jobs is to collect and carry the fluid that has leaked out of the blood vessels back into the circulation through ducts just under the collarbones. If the average adult heart circulates twenty liters[133] of blood daily, about three liters leak out into the spaces between cells (interstitial fluid); this needs to be collected and re-circulated. So, one function of the lymphatic system is as the silent collection partner of the blood vessels. A damaged, pressured, or leaky lymphatic system is often at the root of swelling or edema.

Another role played by the lymphatic system involves immunity. You may notice that when you get a cold or sore throat, the nodes in your neck swell and get a little sore. Those nodes are *lymph nodes*, and they contain large groups of white blood cells. The lymphoid system also includes the *thymus* glands in the upper chest (where white blood cells mature and become ready for action), the *spleen* in the upper left abdomen, the *tonsils* in the back of the throat, the *bone marrow* (which produces white blood cells), and nodes throughout the digestive system and the rest of the body. Lymph nodes tend to cluster at major joints like the front of the hips (inguinal lymph nodes), the backs of the knees, under the armpits, along the spine, and along the neck. This entire network of solid organs and tissues and liquid-carrying vessels is responsible for protecting us from infections.

As if that were not enough, a third part of the lymphatic system (called the lacteal ducts) carries fatty fluids from the intestines through the thoracic duct into the circulation.

Since the lymphatics lack a central pump, what moves the fluid and immune cells through them? Some lymphatic vessels have

---

133 A liter is roughly the same volume as a quart.

their own tiny muscles that squeeze fluid, but for the most part, the lymphatic flow is stimulated by contraction of other muscles. If the lymphatic flow is blocked, there is usually swelling. The best example of this is swollen feet in pregnant women. The baby presses against the lymphatic vessels in the mother's belly, increasing pressure and reducing the flow of lymph in her legs. This leads to swollen feet. Compressing the legs with special stockings or simply raising the legs can usually relieve the pressure and allow the lymph to flow properly, particularly if the mother rests on her left side.

3. The Nervous System

The brain serves as the central command center of the nervous system, and its electrical signals can be roughly measured with an electroencephalogram (EEG)[134]. The spinal cord, running from the brain down the center of the spinal column, sends and receives signals throughout the body through nerves, which send instant messages to each other both electrically and chemically[135]. In addition, the autonomic nervous system (ANS) runs through a series of small networks (mini-brains) and nerves, carrying special information to and from the heart, lungs, digestive system, kidneys, endocrine glands, reproductive organs, the lymphatics, and the skin. The ANS is further divided into the sympathetic nervous system (which generates the fight/flight response) and the parasympathetic nervous system (which generates the rest/digest response). And then there are the special nerves of sensation for our eyes, ears, nose, and taste buds. Whew! Command, control, and communication are complicated.

---

134 Its magnetic signals can be measured with a newer instrument, the magneto-encephalogram (MEG).

135 Chemical messengers for the brain and nerves are called *neurotransmitters*.

The vast majority of the nervous system is involved in unconsciously collecting and analyzing information, interpreting, communicating, and regulating the vast symphony of activity happening every second that keeps us alive. It's not true that we only use 10 percent of our brain. It just that we are generally unaware of 90 percent of what our brain is doing. While you're reading, your brain is ensuring that your last meal is digested; your blood sugar is kept in a certain range, as is your temperature; your heart is beating and lungs are breathing enough to keep oxygen levels proper; your kidneys are filtering blood and maintaining the proper blood sugar; your parathyroid gland is ensuring the right levels of calcium for your cells to contract; and your immune system is maintaining vigilance against nasty foreign invaders while befriending and nurturing the healthy bacteria that help us. Aren't you glad you don't have to think about all of that with your conscious mind? As we learn in medicine, "The dumbest kidney is smarter than the smartest kidney doctor." Not that kidney doctors aren't brilliant. But their conscious minds simply cannot do what the body does every minute without our conscious input.

The glia are the small cells and tissues that surround, protect, insulate, and nourish nerve cells; they also help metabolize neurotransmitters, and they aid in communication among cells and tissues. They used to be considered inert scaffolding and insulation for the nerves. Recently they have been included in the nervous system because they are derived from the same embryonic cells as the nerves and skin, and they carry information. It is said that the more intelligent the species, the higher the ratio of glia to nerve cells in the brain. Einstein had a larger than usual number of glial cells.

I want to emphasize the various nerve plexus centers throughout the body because they roughly correspond to important parts of ancient Ayurvedic anatomy. While the brain is responsible for overall command and control, these mini-brains exercise local authority and interact closely with the endocrine system:

a. The lumbosacral plexus (pelvic mini-brain) contains nerves from the lower part of the spinal cord. It has many branches interacting in the lower abdomen and pelvis; some go on to form the major nerves of the genital organs and legs. This plexus is sometimes divided into two parts (lumbar and sacral), the first of which serves mostly the legs, while the latter serves mostly the genitals, bladder, and anus. It corresponds roughly to the first two chakras (described below) in Ayurvedic functional anatomy.

b. The solar or celiac plexus and the enteric nervous system in the belly involve nerves for the intestinal system, including liver and pancreas, kidneys, adrenal glands, and diaphragm; they roughly correspond to the third Ayurvedic chakra described below. The enteric nervous system (belly mini-brain) does most of the direct regulation of intestinal activity, including moving things along, sensing fullness and composition of meals, communicating with the trillions of bacteria that live in our gut, and regulating blood flow and enzyme release, rates of absorption, and contractions of the gall bladder. Like the brain and its central nervous system, the enteric nervous system uses both electrical and chemical signals. In fact, it uses over thirty different neurotransmitters for communication—in most cases, the same ones used in the brain. Did you know that over 90 percent of the body's serotonin is found in the gut? No wonder when we're nervous we get butterflies in the stomach or when we get sudden bad news we feel as if we've been kicked in the gut. Talk about a mind–body connection!

c. The cardiopulmonary plexus has been discussed above, and corresponds to the fourth Ayurvedic chakra.

d. The brachial plexus in the neck and shoulder sends nerves to the arms and hands. It's associated with minor chakras in the shoulders and hands.

e. The cervical plexus in the throat affects the head, neck, shoulders, thyroid gland, and parathyroid glands, and it corresponds to the fifth chakra.

4. The Endocrine System

This is another anatomic system with close counterparts in ancient Ayurvedic anatomy. While the nervous system communicates electrically and chemically, the endocrine system communicates nearly entirely through chemicals called hormones. Classically, the endocrine system contains the three organs in the brain (pineal, hypothalamus, and pituitary, corresponding to the sixth and seventh chakras), two in the neck (thyroid and parathyroid), two in the abdomen (the pancreas and the two-part adrenal glands, located on top of each kidney), and the reproductive glands. However, in recent years, it has become clear that many organs, including the heart, stomach, intestines, liver, and kidneys, as well as bones, bone marrow, muscle, uterus, placenta, and fat, also release and respond to hormones. This disseminated system forms a vast network that interacts closely with the nervous system, immune system, and many other organs and tissues.

5. The Musculo-Skeletal and Connective Tissue Systems

When someone is mentally or emotionally tense, her muscles are tense. When someone is chronically worried or under pressure, the muscles of her back, neck, arms, and legs are often chronically contracted. Chronically contracted muscles create pain. Muscles also move lymph, and relaxed, flexible muscles are more effective than tight, fixed muscles in doing this job. Relaxing muscle tension is an important goal (and often the most obvious effect) of healing.

The connective tissue surrounds every tissue, organ, and muscle of the body. The connective tissue also connects muscles to bones (tendons). It not only provides protection and a structural framework, but it also supplies the infrastructure and building blocks for the systems for immunity and repair work, and helps relay hormones from their origins to their targets. Furthermore, like the endocrine (hormonal) and nervous systems, the connective tissue system communicates using chemical (such as cytokines and growth factors), electrical, and mechanical signals. In fact, some research suggests that acupuncture works in part through connective tissue signaling[136].

6. The Skin

The skin is the largest and most visible organ in the human body. An enormous amount of communication occurs through human touch, and observant healers can learn a great deal by observing the color, texture, dryness, moisture, wrinkles, folds, rashes, scars, and tension of the skin. In fact, there's a whole field of medicine, dermatology, devoted to the study of skin.

During healing, one indication that someone is becoming relaxed is improved circulation, developing a more rosy skin color. However, be aware that embarrassment, anger, and stress can also lead to a red face, so be sure that you combine observations of the skin along with

---

136 Langevin H.M. , et al., "Mechanical signaling through connective tissue: a mechanism for the therapeutic effect of acupuncture," *FASEB J* 15, no. 12 (2011): 2275–82.
Langevin H.M., "Acupuncture, connective tissue, and peripheral sensory modulation," *Crit Rev Eukaryot Gene Expr* 24,no. 3 (2014): 249–53.

breathing, muscle tension, and verbal information when you make an assessment.

We will skip the digestive, reproductive, breathing, skeletal, and detox (kidney) systems here to turn our attention to two ancient anatomic systems: Ayurveda and Traditional Chinese Medicine (TCM).

Ayurvedic Anatomy: Prana, Nadis, and Chakras

Ayurveda is the traditional medicine of India, which is also practiced in Nepal and other parts of Southeast Asia. Its oral tradition dates back to the fifth century BC. Ayurveda's classical texts were written in Sanskrit over 1,500 years ago, covering general principles, anatomy, embryology, pathology, diagnostics, therapeutics, pharmaceutics, aphrodisiacs, toxicology, obstetrics, pediatrics, ophthalmology, aging, psychiatry, and surgery.

As might be expected in a medical system that included surgery, historical Ayurveda had detailed descriptions of anatomy, including the skin, muscles, joints, bones and bone marrow, heart, lungs, kidneys, liver, spleen, reproductive organs, sensory organs and fluids, such as bile, blood, chyle, phlegm, saliva, semen, and urine[137].

In addition to the concrete concepts of gross anatomy which focus on structure, Ayurveda also includes functional concepts, such as prana. Prana means life force, a universal energy that gives the body heat and life and maintains health. Because it is an ancient system whose origins predate written records, the basis for the concepts of prana and its circulation remain a mystery. It is possible that intuitive observers with long-standing practices of yoga and meditation developed the descriptions of pranic circulation based on

137 Wujastyk D., "A body of knowledge: The Wellcome Ayurvedic Anatomical Main and his Sanskrit Context," *Asian Medicine* no. 4 (2008): 201–48.

their own personal experiences, comparing notes with one another, and eventually codifying the system.

In humans, prana is believed to circulate through three large channels (the Ida, the Pingala, and the Sushumna) and thousands of smaller channels (nadis). The flow of prana continues as long as a person is alive and is considered the ultimate source of life energy that maintains the physical body. Just like Traditional Chinese Medicine has acupoints, Ayurveda has marma points, which serve as doors or entry points to the energetic channels.

Ayurveda: Sushumna, Ida, and Pingala Plus Chakras

For Western health professionals, the easiest way to visualize the three large pranic channels in Ayurveda is to imagine a caduceus. The Sushumna is the central channel running along the spinal column from the bottom, straight up to the brain, ending at the top of the scalp, like the central column of the caduceus. The Ida and Pingala are like the two snakes with their tails starting at the tip of the tailbone. The Ida (carrying the feminine, lunar-type prana) ends at the left nostril and Pingala (carrying the masculine, solar-type prana) ends at the right nostril[138].

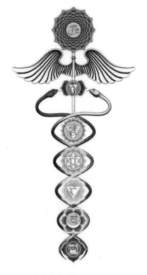

© **Dirk Czarnota**
Fotolia.com

---

138 In some systems, the Ida and Pingala weave back and forth around the Sushumna like the snakes of the caduceus. In other systems, they are thought to travel straight up alongside the Sushumna, in slightly smaller, more flexible columns.

Ayurveda: Chakra Locations

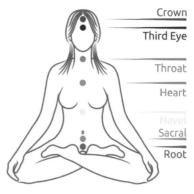

Crown
Third Eye
Throat
Heart
Navel
Sacral
Root

In addition to the nadis carrying prana throughout the subtle or etheric body, there are several pranic vortices, wheels, or whirl-pools (called chakras) along the Sushumna. In some diagrams, the major charkas occur at the top and bottom of the Sushumna and at several points along the way,

© **branchecarica – Fotolia.com**

often corresponding to a major nerve plexus and/or endocrine organ. Because these chakras are part of the functional, subtle, etheric body, they cannot be seen with dissection or surgery, and there is disagreement about their number (varying from five to eight) and how best to represent them (the shape varies from wheels to flowers to cones; colors vary, as well)[139]. One system describes seven chakras, each

---

139 Other texts covering chakras in detail include:

Douglas Baker, M.D., *The Human Aura: A Study of the Human Energy Fields*, (Baker eBooks Publishing, 1986).

Shafica Karagulla, M.D. and Dora van Gelder Kunz, *The Chakras and Human Energy Fields*, (Theosophical Publishing House, 1989).

Brenda Davies, M.D., *The 7 Healing Chakras: Unlocking Your Body's Energy Centers*, (Ulysses Press, 2000).

Anodea Judith, Ph.D., *Wheels of Life*, (Llewellyn Publications, 1987).

Keith Sherwood, *Chakra Therapy for Personal Growth and Healing*, (Llewellyn Publications, 1988).

Barbara Brennan, *Hands of Light: A Guide to Healing Through the Human Energy Field*, (Bantam, 1988).

Rosalyn Bruyere, *Wheels of Light: Chakras, Auras, and the Healing Energy of the Body*, (Fireside Books, 1989).

Cyndi Dale, *The Subtle Body: An Encyclopedia of Your Energetic Anatomy*, (Sounds True, 2009).

Christina Ross, Ph.D., *Etiology: How to Detect Disease in Your Energy Field Before It Manifests in Your Body*, (XLibris, 2013).

CW Leadbetter, *The Chakras*, (Quest Books, 1990).

Chakra Number	Approximate Location in the Physical Body	Associated Color	Associated Nerve Plexus	Associated Endocrine or Other Gland/Organ
7	The crown, at the top, in some cases extending above the top of the head	White or purple	Brain/cerebral cortex	Pineal gland
6	The head, roughly at the level of the pituitary gland, between and slightly above the midpoint of the eyes	Violet or purple or indigo	Brain, mid-brain	Hypothalamus/ pituitary gland
5	The neck, roughly at the level of the thyroid gland	Blue	Cervical plexus	Thyroid and parathyroid glands
4	The chest, roughly at the level of the heart	Green	Cardio-pulmonary plexus	Heart and thymus
3	The upper abdomen, at the solar plexus (this chakra is sometimes divided into two sub-parts, creating eight chakras)	Yellow	Solar or celiac plexus	Adrenals, kidneys, pancreas, liver, stomach
2	The lower abdomen, about a hand's breadth below the navel	Orange	Lumbar plexus	Spleen; bladder
1	The perineum, the originating point of the Sushumna	Red	Sacral plexus	Ovaries and testes; large intestine

associated with a primary color. In addition, many people associate the subtle or etheric chakras with a neural and/or endocrine counterpart:

The systems that describe only five major chakras usually combine the two chakras in the head and the two chakras in the abdomen.

In addition to these major chakras, there are secondary chakras in the palm of each hand and the sole of each foot, and smaller chakras at the major joints.

Different writers and belief systems ascribe various functions to the chakras. There are no empiric studies comparing or evaluating these contrasting numbers of chakras or their precise locations, colors, or functions. However, healers may wish to meditate on, visualize, and imagine these pranic channels and chakras to develop their own intuition and a shared vocabulary and internal experience with other healers.

Traditional Chinese Medicine (TCM) Anatomy

"That feels just like acupuncture without the needles!"

—JOYCE N., AFTER RECEIVING THERAPEUTIC TOUCH TREATMENT

Acupuncture and TCM are also relevant to healers' understanding of anatomy. As with Ayurveda, the history of Traditional Chinese Medicine predates recorded history. TCM healing includes not only acupuncture, but an elaborate herbal repertoire and recommendations about environmental health (feng shui), exercise (Qigong and tai chi), nutrition, social relationships, and massage (tuina).

TCM Meridians

As with Ayurveda's belief in the vital life force, called *prana*, TCM includes belief in a vital life energy known as *qi* (ki in Japan) that circulates through channels, called *meridians* (akin to Ayurveda's nadis). A disruption or imbalance in the flow or amount of qi is associated with poor health, and the healer's job is to help restore the proper flow of qi.

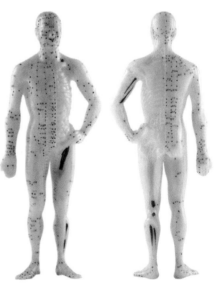

© Unclesam – Fotolia.com

The pattern of flowing qi differs somewhat from the pattern of flowing prana. In TCM, qi flows through fourteen major paired meridians, most of which are associated with the name of a modern anatomical organ, but have functional effects that are not quite the same as that Western biomedical organ. The pairs each include a yin and yang meridian as Chinese Taoist philosophy rests upon the balance of opposites. Most meridians are associated with a fundamental quality or element, and are thought to be most active at specific times of day. Yang meridians tend to run from higher to lower (if the arms are raised), whereas the yin meridians tend to run from lower to higher or from central to peripheral.

A few meridians lack a specific counterpart in terms of Western anatomical organs, and may be thought of metaphorically or functionally. Many of the meridians contain multiple branches, some of which dive below the surface of the body to reach internal organs. They may touch or intersect at the beginning and end of their routes, creating a long, interconnecting set of loops.

Meridian Pair	Location	Most Active Time of Day/Element
Conception (yin) Governing Vessel (yang)	The conception vessel runs from the perineum, up the midline of the front of the body, and to a point below the lower lip. The governing vessel runs from the coccyx, up the midline of the back, and over the head to a point just above the upper middle teeth.	"extra meridians"
Stomach (yang)	The stomach meridian begins at the side of the nose and runs down to the jaw, where it splits. One part runs up in front of the ear to the top of the head. The second part is the main course running from the angle of the jaw to the collar bone, down the chest and belly, the front of the leg, and down to the great toe, where it connects to the beginning of the spleen meridian.	Stomach: 7 to 9 a.m.
Spleen (yin)	The spleen meridian starts at the inside of the great toe and flows upward on the foot and ankle and up the inside of the leg; it zigzags a bit over the abdomen and chest, where part of it enters the body and ascends along the esophagus to the root of the tongue and part continues upward to the space below the second rib, and descends to the armpit and heart area, where it joins the heart meridian.	Spleen: 9 to 11 a.m. Earth

Heart (yin)	The heart meridian starts at the heart, emerges, and spreads from the chest, where it divides into three parts which run: a) upward to just below the eye; b) downward to the small intestine; and c) down the arm to the tip of the little finger, where it links with the start of the small intestine meridian.	Heart: 11 a.m. to 1 p.m.
Small Intestine (yang)	The small intestine meridian starts at the little finger and travels up the arm to the collar bone, where it divides into two branches: a) one heads inward to the small intestine; and b) one goes up the neck and divides, with one part reaching the inner fold of the eye and the other ending just in front of the ear, where it connects with the bladder meridian.	Small intestine: 1 to 3 p.m. Fire
Bladder (yang)	The long bladder meridian runs down the back, the back of the leg, and to the edge of the fifth toe.	Bladder: 3 to 5 p.m.
Kidney (yin)	The kidney meridian starts in the sole of the foot, runs up the inside of the ankle and calf, and on the trunk, ending just under the collarbone.	Kidney: 5 to 7 p.m. Water
Pericardium (yin)	The pericardium meridian starts in the middle of the chest; it splits into three parts: a) one ascends to just below the meeting of the collar bones; b) one descends to just below the navel; and c) the third moves down the arm to the palm side of the long finger.	Pericardium: 7 to 9 p.m.
Triple Warmer or Triple Burner (yang)	The triple burner meridian begins on the pinkie side of the ring finger and runs up the back of the arm, over the collarbone, into the shoulder muscle, and upward behind the ear. One branch turns inward and heads down below the navel; another heads just below the eye; yet another branch enters the ear, emerges in the cheek, and reaches the outer fold of the eye where it meets the gallbladder meridian.	Triple Burner: 9 to 11 p.m. Fire
Gallbladder (yang)	The gallbladder vessel starts at the outer corner of the eye and zigzags over the side and top of the cheek and head before heading down the side of the body all the way to the foot, where it ends on the outside of the great toe and joins the liver meridian.	Gallbladder: 11 p.m. to 1 a.m.
Liver (yin)	The liver meridian starts on the top of the great toe, heads up the leg to the groin, and then zig-zags toward the liver; from the liver, there are two branches: a) one goes up into the lungs where it joins with the lung meridian; b) the other runs up along the throat to the eye (another branch breaks off here and goes to the cheek and lips), emerging in the forehead toward the top of the head where it joins the governing vessel.	Liver: 1 to 3 a.m. Wood

Lung (yin)	The lung meridian starts at the side of the chest near the arm pit, runs down the arm, and ends at the thumbnail.	Lung: 3 to 5 a.m.
Large Intestine (yang)	The large intestine meridian starts at the tip of the pointer finger and runs between the pointer and thumb in the hand, up the arm to the shoulder and neck. It ends between the nose and upper lip to connect with the stomach meridian.	Large Intestine: 5 to 7 a.m. Metal

In addition to the classical acupuncture points (which are similar in Chinese, Japanese, Korean, and French systems of acupuncture, though the specific points may have different names in each language), there are additional systems of lesser meridians and an entire system that relies on acupoints on the ears (auricular acupuncture).

The reason I included the times that each meridian/organ is thought to be most active is that in TCM, the timing of symptoms provides a clue to the involved organ. This is one difference with Western medicine—knowing whether a headache usually occurs at ten a.m. or four p.m. doesn't help much with diagnosis or assessment in Western medicine, but it can be a telling clue in TCM.

What Are the Points Most Often Used in Acupuncture?

Although there are many different points, different systems, and different ways of stimulating points, there is widespread agreement on the value of the "four gates." These four points include two on the hands and two in a similar position on the feet.

Four gates: LI4 (pictured next page)

- Large Intestine 4 (LI4) is located on the back of each hand in the middle of the big muscle between the bones leading to the thumb and first finger. These two points are used for

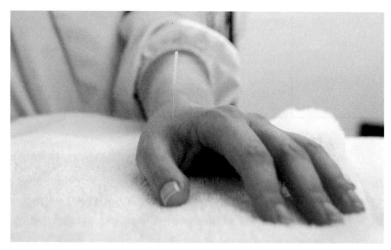

© Tyler Olson – Fotolia.com

many conditions affecting the upper body—headaches, colds, runny nose, sore throat, dizziness, toothaches, sinus pain, nosebleeds, and Bell's palsy. They are also used to help reduce inflammation and pain.

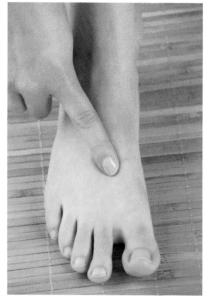

© Monika Wisnewska – Fotolia.com

- Liver 3 (Lv3) is located on the top of the feet in the muscle between the bones leading to the first and second toes, almost like a mirror of Large Intestine 4 points on the hands. This point is used to get things moving and to clear headache and back pain, insomnia, menstrual disorders, emotional problems, and many other conditions.

Four Gates: Lv3

While relatively little scientific research has evaluated the presence and characteristics of Ayurveda's nadis and chakras, abundant scientific research has evaluated acupuncture points.

Can Acupuncture Points Be Detected Reliably?

Yes. A variety of devices have been developed that detect classical acupuncture points and meridian activity by measuring changes in the electrical resistance of the skin[140].

Does Acupuncture Help with Pain?

Yes. Most of the research on acupuncture has evaluated its benefits in treating pain—back pain, headaches, fibromyalgia, abdominal pain, menstrual pain, post-operative pain, and joint pain[141].

---

140 Mayer-Gindner A., et al., "Newly explored electrical properties of normal skin and special skin sites," *Biomed Tech* 49, no. 5 (2004): 117–24. Park H.D., et al., "A new acupuncture point detection using the impedance measurement system based on ANF and phase-space method," *Conf Proc IEEE Eng Med Bio Soc* (2007): 2572–4. Chen C.W., et al., "Wave-induced flow in meridians demonstrated using photoluminescent bioceramic material on acupuncture points," *Evid Based Complement Alternat Med* (2013).

141 Taylor P., et al., "Cost-effectiveness of acupuncture for chronic nonspecific low back pain. *Pain Pract* October 21, 2013). Xu T., et al., "Effects of Moxibustion or Acupoint Therapy for the Treatment of Primary Dysmenorrhea: A Meta-analysis," *Altern Ther Health Med* 20, no. 4 (2014): 33–42. Manyanga T., et al., "Pain management with acupuncture in osteoarthritis: a systematic review and meta-analysis," *BMC Complement Altern Med* 14, no. 1 (2014): 312. Deare J.C., et al., "Acupuncture for treating fibromyalgia," *Cochrane Database Syst Rev*, (May 31, 2013): 5.

How Does Acupuncture Work?

Several studies show that acupuncture treatments help release the body's own internal pain-relieving compounds (endorphins). However, that may not be the whole explanation, since acupuncture can do so many other things that we don't attribute to endorphins, like relieving nausea[142], stimulating ovulation[143], relieving hot flashes[144], and helping turn breech babies around[145]. More research is needed to understand how acupuncture achieves its diverse functional effects.

Although acupuncture's tiny needles are the most well-known way to stimulate acupoints, there are several additional classical methods for stimulating these points—heat (moxibustion), cupping (suction), vigorous massage, tapping, needles plus electrical stimulation, and medical Qigong, in which the healer transmits his own qi to the patient through his hands. Furthermore, different schools of acupuncture may use different points to treat patients with similar conditions. The fact that there are so many different acupoints and that they can be stimulated in so many different ways casts doubt on the usefulness of research using "sham" acupuncture stimulation. Many of the studies using "sham" stimulation have had similar effects to "real" stimulation using needles[146], both of which are superior to

---

142 Cheong K.B., et al., "The effectiveness of acupuncture in prevention and treatment of postoperative nausea and vomiting—a systematic review and meta-analysis," *PLoS One* 8, no. 12 (2013): e82474.

143 Johansson J., et al., "Acupuncture for ovulation induction in polycystic ovary syndrome: a randomized controlled trial," *Am J Physiol Endocrin Metab* 304, no. 9 (2013): E934–43.

144 Chiu H.Y., et al., "Effects of acupuncture on menopause-related symptoms and quality of life in women on natural menopause: a meta-analysis of randomized controlled trials," *Menopause* (July 7, 2014).

145 Coyle M.E., et al., "Cephalic version by moxibustion for breech presentation," *Cochrane Database Syst Rev* (May 16, 2012) 5: CD003928.

146 Pastore L.M., et al., "True and sham acupuncture produced similar frequency of ovulation and improved LH to FSH ratios in women with polycystic ovary syndrome," *J Clin Endocrinol Metab* 96, no. 10 (2011): 143–50.

non-treatment[147]. This suggests that non-needle techniques can be just as effective for many conditions as needle-based treatments.

What Does This Mean for Healers?

If non-needle or sham acupuncture is as effective as true acupuncture, this may imply that one of the critical factors in effectiveness involves the healer–patient relationship, and particularly the healer's ability to communicate being calm and confident and holding the clear, focused intention to relieve suffering. It is also possible that subtle changes in electrical signals in the healer's electromagnetic field are detected in the recipient's connective tissue and then amplified and disseminated, resulting in meaningful clinical improvements. In any case, it may be worthwhile for healers to study and meditate on the traditional meridians to develop their intuition about points and pathways to employ in their healing work. See if you can sense what the first humans who developed acupuncture sensed. Are your senses as keen as ancient acupuncturists or the modern electrical devices used to locate acupoints?

Auras, Etheric, Astral, Mental, and Other Bodies: Theosophical Perspective

Many healers report the ability to see lights or colors that surround and seem to emanate from the physical body, and these "second bodies" are generally called auras[148].

---

147 Vas J., "Acupuncture in patients with acute low back pain: a multicenter randomized controlled clinical trial," *Pain* 153, no. 9 (2012): 1883–9.

148 D.M. Baker, *The Human Aura: A Study of Human Energy Fields*, (1986).

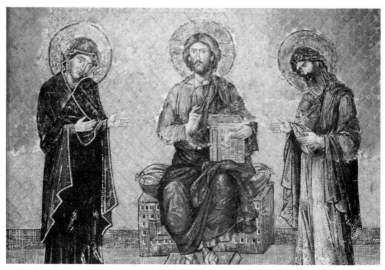

© Senai Aksoy – Fotolia.com

Christian Image of Auras

The most familiar example of this in Western art is the halo. This halo (or aura) is referred to by theosophists C.W. Leadbetter[149] , Dora van Gelder Kunz[150], and Rudolph Steiner, the founder of Anthroposophy, as the *etheric body*; others call it the *vital body*.

The etheric body (or aura) is closely related to physical vitality. This biofield was detected in a series of experiments by Dr. Walter Kilner, using special screens and filters in a series of experiments at the turn of the last century[151]. The etheric body, and all the layers of the aura, overlap with the physical body and extend beyond the skin.

The next, more subtle aura, extending slightly farther out, is the *astral body*, which is usually associated with emotional states and patterns.

---

149 C.W. Leadbetter, *Man, Visible and Invisible, 2nd edition*, (Quest Books, 2000).
150 Dora van Gelder Kunz, *The Personal Aura*, (Quest Books, 1991).
151 Walter Kilner, *The Human Aura*, (University Books, 1965).

Even finer and more expansive than the astral is the *mental body*, which connects us with the minds of all others, the collective mind, or unconscious archetypes. This is thought to be the level where brilliant insights or intuitions arise. The *spiritual body* connects humans with the creative spirit or energy of the Universe; this is the most subtle and largest of the human auras.

Layers of the Human Body: Etheric, Astral, Mental, and Spiritual Body with Chakras

Chakras and auras are part of the functional anatomic understanding of several healing systems and traditions, including the Cherokee, Egyptian, Incan, and shamanic systems around the world.

Try sensing these different kinds of auras or subtle bodies yourself. It is not necessary to sense them in order to be helpful, but you may find it interesting to experience what others have reported.

Plant and Mineral Anatomy

Just as ancient health care systems viewed humans as having prana and qi, these life forces (or subtle energies) have also been attributed to animals, plants, minerals, and places. In homeopathy and similar systems, this unique life force or subtle energy can be amplified by a process of repeatedly diluting and shaking the original substance in pure water. In many cases, no molecules of the original substance remain in the water, but the energy/information is thought to be more potent. This is a belief system that is hard to reconcile with modern notions of biochemistry, but it is an interesting exercise for healers to sit quietly with a tree or an herb, and in the stillness, attune more closely to the healing properties that may be found there. What will you find?

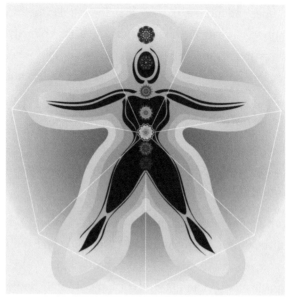

© artellia – Fotolia.com

Now that we've thoroughly prepared ourselves physically, mentally, and spiritually, and have reviewed conventional and ancient anatomy, let's get going with some healing practices, strategies, and techniques. That's what Part 3 is all about.

Step-by-Step Guide to Healing Practices, Strategies, and Techniques

CHAPTER 11

Warm-up Exercises

We have completed the basics of setting an intention; undertaken physical, emotional, mental, and spiritual preparation; and learned about the basic anatomical systems involved in healing work. Now it's time to move into some warm-up exercises before we launch into actual healing practices. This is where it gets fun! It's even more fun to find a practice partner so you can compare notes. Remember, these are warm-ups. You are not being graded, and there is no right or wrong answer. Just enjoy the process. Plan, act, observe, reflect, repeat.

There are ten warm-up exercises in this chapter. You do not have to do them all at once. Take your time. The important thing is to observe what you are sensing without judgment as you do each exercise. Feel free to do one a day or one a week, some alone and some with a friend, family member, or colleague. This is a learning adventure. Enjoy.

Warm-up Exercise #1: What's Between My Hands?

The first warm-up practice that beginning healers do to start to develop their sense of touch is to notice what's between their hands at different distances. Sitting or standing upright with your feet flat on the floor, hold your hands in front of you, palms lightly pressed together as if in prayer or the "Namaste" in yoga.

1. Start by rubbing your hands together vigorously for 15 to 30 seconds to warm them up.
2. Now move your hands about 12 inches (30 centimeters) apart with palms facing each other. What do you notice?
3. Slowly, move them to within 1/2 inch (1 cm) of each other.
4. Now separate them about 6 inches (15 cm) and then narrow the gap to 2 to 3 inches (7 cm).
5. Note what you feel between your hands at each distance in a practice journal.

Warm-up #1: What's Between my Hands?

Repeat this process of rubbing your hands together and bouncing them farther apart. Try 18 inches, 3 feet, as far apart as you can stretch, and then move them in closer, palms facing each other until your hands nearly touch. Try it with your eyes open and again with your eyes closed. What do you notice in the space between your hands? Do you feel it more strongly in the fingertips or the palms?

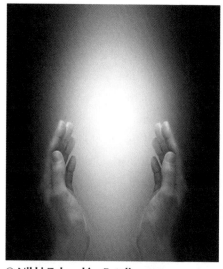

© Nikki Zalewski – Fotolia.com

Hands at Different Distances Apart from Each Other

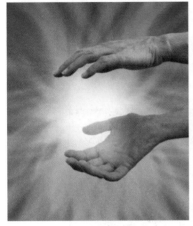 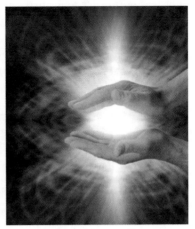

© Nikki Zalewski – Fotolia.com   © Nikki Zalewski – Fotolia.com

There are no right or wrong answers. Many people notice a sense of fullness, tingling, pulsing, magnetism, or heat between their hands, most often in the middle of the palm. Some people describe it as "energy." For most folks, there is a sense of slight resistance as the hands get closer and sense of stretching or elasticity as they move farther apart—almost as if there is some kind of very light taffy between the hands that stretches and compresses as the hands move farther apart and closer together.

Warm-up Exercise # 1 Variation

This time as you move your hands closer and farther away, try moving them slightly off-center as if you were exploring a light, flexible ball between your hands about 6 inches (15 cm) in diameter. As you explore the dimensions and qualities of this object, notice whether it seems larger or smaller than the 6-inch diameter. Can you compress or stretch it? Is it round or oval? What else do you notice? Don't worry if you don't feel anything. You can still try the other warm-up exercises[152].

Warm-up Exercise #1 Variation: Rolling an Imaginary Ball between Your Hands

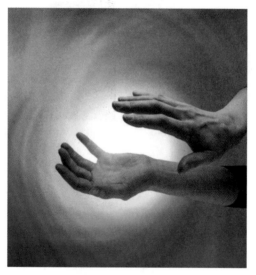

© Nikki Zalewski – Fotolia.com

Warm-up Exercise #2: What's around My Arms and Legs?

For the second warm-up, let's see if the feeling we noticed between our hands is present on our arms and legs. If you're right-handed, start out using your right hand. If you're left-handed, use the left. Sit-

---

152 There is nothing wrong with you if you can't feel anything with these exercises right away. I couldn't see anything besides my eyelashes the first few times I looked in a microscope. This didn't mean there was anything wrong with me or my equipment; it sometimes takes a while to get used to seeing something in a new way. Be patient with yourself and the process of discovery.

ting upright with your feet flat on the floor, hold your hands in front of you, palms lightly pressed together.

1. Rub your hands together for 15 to 30 seconds.
2. Take your right hand and hold it about 3 to 6 inches (7 to 15 cm) over your left shoulder and bounce your hand gently closer and farther over the shoulder until it settles at a comfortable distance from the shoulder.
3. Run the right hand from the shoulder down the arm, over the elbow, down the forearm, the wrist, and out to the fingers.
4. Repeat this 3 to 6 times at different *speeds* and *different distances* from your left arm, noticing the sensations in both your right hand and your left arm as you do.
5. Stop. Hold your right hand, palm up, in your lap. How does it feel?
6. Wash your hands in lukewarm water. How does your right hand feel after washing and drying your hands?

Warm-up Exercise #2 Variations

a. Use your left (non-dominant) hand over your right shoulder and arm.
b. Run your right hand over the top of your right leg from your hip to the top of your toes. Switch to the left hand over the left leg.
c. Cross over. Run the right hand over the left leg and vice versa.
d. Both hands together. Run the right hand over the right leg while running the left hand over the left leg.

What do you notice when you compare the different variations? Note that in your practice journal.

If you've ever gone to a wine-tasting event, you know that you "cleanse your palate" between trying different kinds of wine. Some people drink a sip of water. Some eat a plain cracker. Some take a bite of cheese. Different approaches have slightly different effects on the taste of the next glass of wine.

Try "cleansing" your hands between each variation in one of three ways:

1. Wash them in tepid water.
2. Shake your hands out vigorously as if flicking off ants that had crawled on them at a picnic.
3. Put both hands on the ground for a few seconds.

What do you notice? Many people find that when they run their hands slightly above the body, they sense a buildup of static or stickiness. This static or stickiness can be removed by gently washing, flicking, or "grounding" the hands. Is that your experience?

If you don't feel anything, that's fine. If you notice something different than what someone else notices, that's fine, too. Keep notes in your practice journal so you can reflect on these experiences later on your own or with a practice buddy or teacher.

Next let's try some practices in which your hands are physically touching part of your body rather than hovering over it.

Warm-up Exercise #3: Muscles vs. Joints

If you've looked at any of the anatomical acupuncture dolls, you may have noticed that acupuncture points tend to occur in bunches over joints, while they are more scattered over large muscles. Why is that? Let's find out.

Feel free to take a break between any steps to note what you observe in your practice journal. Also feel free to wash, flick, or ground your hands between any steps.

1. Take a few deep, slow breaths to calm yourself and enter the peaceful part of yourself in which you are quiet and can easily hear, see, and pay attention as a neutral observer.

2. Place your hands over the large muscles in the front of your thighs, right hand on right thigh, and left hand on left thigh. Leave them there about 30 seconds. What do you notice? Now move both hands to one thigh, side by side. Again, hold for about 30 seconds and note the sensations in your hands and your thighs.

3. Lean over and put one hand on your shin and the other on the calf of the same leg, cradling your lower leg between your hands. Try not to let your hands touch each other. Hold them there about 30 seconds. How does that compare with holding both hands on the same thigh? Do you feel a connection between your hands through your leg?

4. Put one hand over your knee and the other hand over the ankle of the same leg. You can move them around to see if it feels better to hold the front of the knee (kneecap) or the back or sides of the knee and the same with the ankle. Try not to cross your legs. There is not a "right" way, but there are more and less comfortable ways of doing this. Hold them there about 30 seconds. Do you feel a connection between your hands? What is the feeling like in your shin and calf muscles?

5. Switch the hands, so the hand that was on the knee is now on the ankle, and the hand that was on the ankle is now on the knee. Again, move them around so they're comfortable. Hold them there about 30 seconds. Do you feel a connection between your hands? What is the feeling like in your shin and calf muscles? How does it compare to the feeling in your hands and legs in step 4?
6. Repeat steps 4 and 5 using the other leg. How does it compare to the first leg?

One purpose of this exercise is to compare the sense of connection in your hands between hands over muscle versus hands over joints. Most people feel the sense of connection more easily when their hands are over joints; the normal tension in muscles can feel almost like armor or a shield, preventing you from sensing more deeply.

As you start to sense the connection between your hands when they are both on the body, you may also notice that one hand is dominant (feels like it's sending) and the other is more receptive. You're likely to notice this most when they are separated a bit, as when one is over the knee and the other is over the ankle. The hand you usually use for writing and throwing tends to be the dominant one in healing, but not always.

Another thing to notice in this exercise is the difference between having your hands side by side (as they were over the thigh) versus on the front and back of the body (as on the shins and calves). For this comparison, pay more attention to the feeling in the legs than the feeling in the hands. Most people sense things more deeply when the hands are cradling a part of the body like a sandwich than when the hands are side by side. What's your experience? Everyone is a little different, but repeating these exercises with others and talking about it together will help you get a sense of what it feels like from the recipient's standpoint.

Warm-up Exercise #4: Compare Right and Left Side of Body

In the last exercise, we started by placing hands on thighs. This is a good introduction to the next exercise in which we will compare sensations on the right and left sides of the body. It is important when doing these exercises to remember that most of us have dominant and non-dominant hands. Just as it's easier to write or throw with one hand, you may notice that it's easier to sense things with one hand, and that the sensations (or your interpretation of sensations) may differ in your dominant and non-dominant hand.

Why is this important? If you tend to feel things are "warmer" in your left hand, you may attribute the warmth to the person you are working with and misattribute the warmth (interpreting it as inflammation or increased blood flow or pain) to the recipient instead of your own side-to-side differences. So, before you start assessing or helping someone else, get to know yourself well with these exercises.

1. Start by putting your hands on each foot at the same time—right hand on top of the right foot; left hand in the same position on top of the left foot. Rest them there about 15 seconds, comparing the sensations in your hands, noticing whether you are most sensitive to sensations in your fingertips, fingers, or palms.
2. Shift your hands up to your shins—right hand to right shin and left hand to left shin. Repeat your observations, comparing sensations in the left and right hands.

3. Move your hands up to the thighs. Repeat this process all the way up to the top of your head.

4. Take a minute to note your observations in your practice journal. Does one hand usually feel warmer or colder, more tingly, sticky, full, or prickly than the other? Or are they exactly the same? Are they the same over the legs, but different over the head? As you move your hands, notice whether there is a breeze in the room or sunlight or a heater on one part of the body that might affect the temperature.

5. Repeat the sequence, but instead of having both hands on the body at once, alternate them so that each hand has a chance to feel the same leg, the same side of the belly, the same side of the head. How does that differ from having hands on opposite sides at the same time? Again, take a minute to note your observations in your practice journal. If you are working with someone else, this is a great time to compare notes.

Warm-up Exercise #5: Compare the Inner and Outer Sides of the Arms and Legs, Hands and Feet.

Since the inner legs are nearer to each other, they tend to be warmer than the outer part of the legs. Similarly, the inner parts of the arms are closer to the body and tend to be warmer than the outer parts of the arms. Take a moment to compare the sensations. For example, the inner side of the knees (where they'd touch if holding the legs together) compared to the opposite, outer side of the knees. Try the same thing with the inside of the elbow (where one part of the arm touches another as you bend your arm) to the outside of the elbow; the inner wrist to the outer wrist; and the palm to the back of the hand. What do you notice? Note your observations in your practice journal.

Warm-up Exercise #6: Compare Same Side to Opposite Sides

This time we'll pay attention to what it feels like where our hands are touching rather than in the hands themselves. This will help us be more empathetic to those we are trying to help later on.

1. Put the right hand on the right knee and left hand on the left hip. Note the sensation in the knee and hip. What do you notice when your hands are on opposite sides of the body? Switch hands. How do the sensations change in the knee and hip?

2. Repeat the same exercise with the left hand to left knee and right hand to left shoulder (same side of the body). Switch to the right side of the body. How does this compare to when your hands were on opposite sides of the body?

It's a little awkward to do these exercises on yourself, but it's the most convenient and easiest way to get started. If you have a practice buddy, try these exercises on each other and give each other feedback. The main thing here is to start to become more sensitive to the sensations in your hands and how different hand positions (same or opposite sides of the body) feel to the part being touched.

"You can see a lot by just looking."

—YOGI BERRA

You can learn to sense a lot more with your hands by touching, too. And touching in different places, in different combinations, and with varying pressure can enhance your sensitivity as well as help you empathize with a recipient.

In the first two exercises, we practiced sensing the space between our hands and over our arms. Let's return to practices that increase our awareness and ability to sense things beyond the visible edge of the skin. If you've ever been with someone else in a cold place, you may have moved closer to share some warmth. We know that our body heat doesn't stop at our skin. Let's do some testing to see just how far away from the skin we can sense that heat.

Warm-up Exercise #7: Hands at Different Distances from the Skin

Start by sitting up in a comfortable position and taking a few breaths to return to the peaceful, quiet, neutral, curious place within you. Even if you've done this exercise before, you might be surprised at what you observe THIS time.

1. Review the directions from warm-up exercise 1. Rub your hands together for a few seconds to warm them up, and then move them apart and together slowly so you can sense them without touching.

2. With your dominant hand, pick an easy place to reach (belly or thigh, for example), and see if you can sense how far away from your skin you can feel the heat and other signals emanating from your body. For example, if your hand is on your thigh, you might be able to notice the tension in the muscle, even under a pair of pants and layers of skin.

3. Can you continue to sense it as your hand moves 1/2 inch away from direct contact? What about 2 inches? And so

on. If your hand is on your belly, you might be able to feel it rumbling, and you can probably feel your breathing as you breathe in and out. Can you continue to sense those dynamic sensations as you gently move your hand away from direct contact? You may be surprised that some sensations are actually easier to detect with a very light touch or being a few inches away from direct contact. Or you may not feel anything other than the body's radiant heat.

How do you think those sensations would change if your thigh muscle had just been exercising doing lunges or deep knee bends? How might they change if you'd just walked in from the cold or sat in front of a fire?

There are no wrong observations; there is just learning from what you observe. Do not force yourself into imagining what you think you should be feeling. In order to learn from these experiences, it is best to be honest with yourself.

For the last three exercises, we will transition from the hands being relatively still to being in motion.

Warm-up Exercise #8: Hands Still vs. Hands Moving

This is an opportunity to notice the different sensations in your hands when they are still compared with when they are moving. To minimize the distraction of comparing the textures of different materials (bare skin versus cotton jeans versus silk shirt versus corduroy skirt), let's do these exercises with the hands about 1 to 6 inches from the body. You should be close enough that you can still feel some heat emanating from the body, but not so close that you'll be in direct contact. It's a bit like standing in line—not so close that you crowd the person in front of you, and not so far apart that someone else cuts in front of you.

1. Start by sitting up in a comfortable position and taking a few breaths to return to the peaceful, quiet, neutral, curious place within you.

2. Place your dominant hand slightly above your other shoulder. Just hold it there for several seconds, noting the temperature, the sense of whether the muscles are tight or relaxed, and anything else that seems interesting.

3. While keeping the hand about the same distance away from the body, move the hand up toward the ear, and then gradually sweep it downward toward the elbow. The purpose here is to compare your sense of the shoulder when your hand hovers in stillness over it to your sense of it as you move across it from ear to elbow. It may help to repeat the sweeping motion several times. Then try one more time just hovering the hand over the shoulder. Note your observations in your practice journal.

4. Repeat the same activity with your non-dominant hand and your other shoulder, noting your observations in your journal. Were there differences in the right and left sides? What was the feeling in your shoulders with the hand hovering versus sweeping?

5. Repeat this activity with your dominant hand over the opposite thigh (a muscle instead of a joint). Hover over it for a bit, and then sweep your hand from the hip to the knee over the thigh. Try it with the non-dominant hand over the other thigh. Were there differences from right to left? Were there different sensations in your thigh with hovering versus

sweeping? How did sensations differ as you swept over joints compared to sweeping over muscles?

Some people find a greater sense of connection with hands still than hands moving. In other situations, the experience of hovering (still) hands feels uncomfortable and stuck, whereas moving gives a more pleasurable sense of flowing. Moving hands can convey a sense of clearing out whatever is "stuck" or sluggish, while still hands convey a sense of "filling up" an area of emptiness or "warming" a cool, depleted area.

If you don't feel any difference, that's okay, too. Be kind and patient with yourself as you try these different exercises. Remember, my experience is not the same as your experience. My perception is not necessarily "right" just because I'm writing about it. Discover what is true for you.

Warm-up Exercise #9: Goldilocks—Hands Moving Quickly, Medium, and Slowly

Remember, Goldilocks was on her third bed before she found one that was "just right." For this exercise, please focus on what it feels like in your arm or leg as your hands move over them at different speeds.

1. Start by sitting up in a comfortable position and taking a few breaths to return to the peaceful, quiet, neutral, curious place within you.
2. Using your dominant hand, slowly sweep it over your other arm from shoulder to fingertips. Do this 3 times as slowly as you can. Note the sensation in your arm.
3. Next, sweep your hand over the arm fast, faster, faster! Again, what is that like in your arm?

4. Finally, pick a middle speed and sweep the dominant hand over the opposite arm three times. What did you notice in your arm? What felt the best to you? What do you think would feel best if you were a child? An elderly person? Someone who was in pain or afraid?

5. Repeat this exercise with your non-dominant hand, and try doing it over your legs, as well. If you have a practice partner, this is a fun opportunity to give feedback.

What's the right speed to sweep your hand? It depends. I usually imagine I'm petting a dog or a cat. If you're feeling playful, you may move more quickly than if you are settling down for a nap. An older animal may appreciate a slower pace than a puppy or kitten. Similarly, a sick or frail animal generally prefers slower movements than a robust, healthy pet.

Remember, you can use one of the three "cleansing" techniques between any exercise or even between the steps of an exercise. In health care, it's a good idea to wash hands frequently. If you're practicing at home or with a family member, you can flick your hands or touch the ground or wash hands between exercises.

Warm-up Exercise #10: Moving from High to Low vs. Low to High; Moving Inward vs. Outward

In this exercise we'll compare the sensations we experience as we move our hands in different directions—top to bottom versus feet to head, and center to sides versus sides to center.

1. Start by sitting up in a comfortable position and taking a few breaths to return to the peaceful, quiet, neutral, curious place within you.

2. With your dominant hand over your shoulder, sweep downward at a pace that feels comfortable for you all the way down to your fingertips of the opposite hand. Repeat twice. Notice how that feels in your arm and in your sweeping, sensing hand.

3. The next time, start at your fingertips and sweep upward toward the shoulder or hip. This may feel awkward since most of our sweeps have been downward, so repeat three times.

4. Switch sensing hands. Use your non-dominant hand to sweep downward three times from shoulder to fingertip, and then upward three times. Note your observations in your practice journal. How did the sensations and overall experience differ between downward and upward sweeping?

5. Finally, put your hands in front of your face with your palms facing your face. Sweep the hands outward toward the ears. Then move them down to the front of the neck, and sweep out to the side of the neck. Repeat over the chest, belly, and hips, sweeping from the center (midline) to the sides, outward.

6. Reverse directions. Start with your hands over the sides of your hips (over your holster, you gunslinger), sweeping toward the middle. Repeat the sweeping from the side to the front-center of your body, each time moving a little higher until at least you make a sweep from your ears to the top of your head.

7. Compare the sensations in your body as you swept from center outward and from your sides inward. Which felt more comfortable? More calming? More energizing?

Just as the pace of sweeping can vary depending on the situation, so does the direction of the sweep. For most sick or injured people, slower is better than faster; top to bottom is more soothing than bottom to top; and sweeping from center outward is more comfortable than moving from periphery to center. Again, imagine you're petting a dog or cat. Very few of them like being petted from tail to head. It just goes against the grain, so to speak. In living beings, there are always exceptions to these general rules. Trust your growing intuition, and practice with a partner (or two or three) so you can get plenty of feedback before you start working with someone who is suffering. Practice makes you more confident and calm.

The next few chapters give guidance about helping with common symptoms (stress, fatigue, pain, and nausea), but if you have read all the earlier chapters and have done the suggested exercises, you have already learned the most important thing: remain centered and grounded, and extend loving-kindness and compassion without judgment or attachment. Whether your hands are still or moving, touching or off the body, sweeping up, down, or sideways is much less important than what you do with your heart and mind, your attention and intention. In the next chapter, we'll learn and practice strategies that help promote calm and serenity strategies that help reduce stress.

CHAPTER 12
Calming and Relieving Stress

WHETHER THEY ARE TODDLERS with cuts and bruises, mothers who have miscarried, men with chronic back pain, or anyone living with cancer, heart disease, or AIDS, the vast majority of people who seek healing are stressed and worried. One of the first things I learned when I started studying stress and illness back in the 1970s is that chronic stress makes most all symptoms worse. We did a small study showing that when they'd experienced stressful life events, people with diabetes had higher blood sugars than when their lives were calmer and less stressful. That study was one of the things that sparked my interest in healing and my curiosity to do research—if stress makes things worse, can decreasing stress make it better? Yes!

Stress has powerful, pernicious effects on the brain, immune system, and other bodily systems. It makes us more aware of pain and less able to sleep. And often, stress and its consequences turn into a vicious circle: more stress, more pain, poorer sleep, fatigue, poor immune function, more illness, more stress, more pain, poorer sleep, and so on. Nearly every day, healers have an opportunity to turn this vicious cycle into a virtuous cycle. We can offer a sense of calm and comfort to help someone relax. Feeling calmer and more confident makes it easier to cope and easier to recover, and it helps us more easily rise to the next challenge we face. Even if healers do nothing else, helping someone feel calmer, more confident, more secure, and less stressed and lonely is an incredibly valuable gift.

Negative Emotions Reflect Unmet Needs

When someone expresses anger, anxiety, sadness, stress, worry, or overwhelmed feelings, they are signaling us that their needs are not being met. Negative emotions can be seen as gifts rather than something to avoid, ignore, or fight IF we use them to gain deeper understanding and a wiser approach to serving someone in need.

Although the sound of an alarm clock may be unpleasant, it helps us get up on time. Similarly, negative emotions, though unpleasant, can help us understand and achieve our goal of serving others. Unplugging or silencing an alarm clock may make our mornings more pleasant in the short run, but it impairs our ability to achieve our goals for timeliness. Similarly, responding to others' negative emotions with bland reassurance, blame, or denial may feel temporarily better, but it can create unintended consequences.

So, How Do We Help Someone Feel Calmer and Less Stressed?

Here are three simple tips:

1. Remember you are here to be helpful.
2. Remember to stay centered and grounded in your intention and the peaceful, calm place within you.
3. Offer to help.

Weak Strategies to Manage Negative Emotions and Unintended Consequences

Weak Strategy	Unintended Consequences
Bland reassurance without taking time to fully understand situation	Recipient may see healer as paternalistic and clueless about the extent of the problem.
Empathy alone without compassionate desire to relieve suffering	Recipient may get "stuck" in negative emotions. Healer can pick up stress and become more stressed herself.
"Relax!" "Calm down!" or "should" statements (You should try to get some rest.)	May create resistance by recipient who feels they have every right to their current emotional state and that we simply don't understand them, increasing stress and decreasing trust. Giving orders often increases resistance.
Ignore suffering to focus on fixable medical problems	Patient may feel they are no more than their medical problem, dehumanized, and isolated.
Blaming: "You brought this on yourself by rushing out in the street without looking both ways."	Leads to feeling guilty and less able to make changes or do things that bring relief. Pre-occupation with the past and what might have been rather than what's possible in the moment.

How to Offer to Help

We have covered centering and grounding in great detail previously. Now it's time to talk about how we offer to help.

If someone knows what you can do and asks you to do it, wash your hands and do it. If someone doesn't know what you do, and looks like he's stressed or worried, you might *ask him how he's doing.* It's better to start with an open-ended question, because we really don't know how another person is feeling. We might guess how we would feel in a similar situation, but we can't know for sure if we're not in their shoes.

If you've ever taken a CPR class, you know that before you start doing chest compressions or breathing for someone, you ask "Annie, Annie, are you all right?" If there's no response and it looks like she isn't breathing, you check for breathing and a pulse. Even in an emergency, ask first. And if you don't get a response, look carefully before you leap in. You don't want to disturb someone who is sleeping contentedly.

Let's take a closer look at the "look carefully" advice. One of your most important roles is to observe without judging. As a healer, it is not your role to diagnose disease. By law, that role is confined to selected licensed health professionals. And even for those of us who have that legal right, it is always wise to observe carefully. So, observe carefully—skin color, breathing patterns, posture, activity level (quiet or restless), facial expression, hand movements, tone and pitch of voice, and the presence of any devices or equipment (wheelchair, cane, intravenous line, etc.). Also note whether this person has another person with him—a friend, family member, or a health professional—and whether that person is tending to him already.

If the person says he is stressed or worried, I offer to help using something that:

a. Has helped many people feel calmer and more relaxed and confident
b. Is safe
c. Doesn't require any needles or taking clothes off or anything else uncomfortable
d. Can be stopped whenever they say. It's up to them.

If he declines, saying he's "fine," you have some choices. You can say okay and walk away. Or you can acknowledge what he said and compliment him on coping so well with a situation that many would find stressful. You can tell him you're happy to hear he's fine and to let you know if he feels stressed or worried because you can help with that. If you observe signs of severe stress (e.g., crying, twisting a handkerchief, yelling at someone), you can say what you see (without interpreting or labeling it) and ask if you can help. If the offer is declined, extend goodwill and leave it at that. It is disrespectful (and many would say unethical) to proceed with a healing treatment without permission unless a) it's an emergency; or b) the recipient is incapacitated or unable to give permission but his spouse, parent, or someone else who has health care power of attorney gives you permission.

After you have permission, describe what you are going to do, and wash your hands. It is very helpful for people to have a sense of control and to be able to anticipate what's going to happen. Give as many choices as possible. Would he prefer to sit up or lie down? Would he prefer to have his eyes open or closed? This treatment generally involves some light touch, but it can be done without touching; ask permission before you use a treatment involving touch. Would he like to start at the feet or head? Ask him if he can give a number from zero to ten to describe his stress level (or relaxation level if you prefer to focus on the positive) before you start, and ask him what he would like that level to be by the end of the session. Asking this helps provide an anchor and sets an expectation that stress can (and probably will) decrease. Setting a goal is the first step in accomplishing it. Having choices is empowering and often starts the process of helping someone feel calmer as he realizes how much control he actually has.

Five-Step Summary for Typical Healing Session

There are five basic steps for any healing session:

1. *Center* on the stillness, peace, and harmony within. You can use any of the preparatory practices we covered earlier,

such as visualizing a peaceful place in nature, repeating a positive word, meditating, or prayer. Maintain that center throughout all other steps. Mentally and emotionally *ground* yourself in compassion, extending peace and goodwill to the recipient (May you be safe, secure, comfortable, happy, peaceful, free, etc.). Establish a positive connection by resting your hands lightly on his shoulders (if he's sitting up) or gently holding his feet (if he's reclining) for several seconds or up to a minute.

2. *Observe* the recipient using your eyes, ears, and hands. This is where your warm-up exercise practice will be useful. You can lightly touch the person on the right and left side of the body in front and back (if they can be easily reached), or you can sweep your hands over the body about two to six inches above the skin from head to toe. You may sense an area of greater heat or coolness, fullness or emptiness, tingling, sharp, smooth, or something else. This observation and assessment is NOT diagnosis; it is open, non-judgmental, kind, caring awareness. Remain centered and grounded throughout this step, and continue to be observant throughout the next steps. (More on this step below.) After you assess, develop a plan to restore balance, harmony, and a sense of calm ease.

3. Use your hands either gently on or slightly off the body, either still or moving to help restore a sense of balance, order, and an easy flow throughout the body. We'll talk more about this below.

4. When you feel finished, carefully observe from head to toe using your eyes, ears, and hands in an attitude of curious, accepting, non-judgmental, non-attachment to results.

5. Finish by refocusing on your inner sense of peace and
   harmony. Tell the recipient softly that you are finished, and
   ask how he is feeling now. If he's still awake and can answer
   (many people fall asleep during a healing session), ask if
   he can give another number from zero to ten for his stress
   level now. Wash your hands. If you are working in a health
   care setting, either note your observations in the health
   record or tell someone what you observed and did so she
   can note it in the record. If you are not working in a health
   care setting, write your own notes in your practice journal.
   Include the recipient's pre- and post-session stress levels.
   Health professionals refer to this as a "numeric rating scale,"
   NRS, and it's widely used as a measure of the impact of an
   intervention. The most important part of step 5 is returning to
   your inner sense of peace, harmony, and compassion, and
   allowing the healing process to occur in the recipient. His or
   her healing is out of your hands now.

Now that we have an overview of the 5 steps, which do you think
is most important? Most beginners focus on steps 3 and 4, but the
truth is, the most important steps are preparation and steps 1 and 5.
Since we've already covered the basics of steps 1 and 5 in previous
chapters, we'll focus on steps 2, 3, and 4 here.

Step 2: Observation and Assessment

In the observation and assessment step, you maintain your sense of
being centered and grounded, experiencing and extending a sense of
peacefulness while you kindly and perceptively observe the patient.
Most people who teach healing focus on developing your intuition

with this step, increasing your sensitivity to perceive beyond the anatomically obvious. While it can be very useful to develop your intuition, do not overlook the obvious. And don't be afraid to ask the recipient for feedback.

One time during a Therapeutic Touch workshop, I was working with a middle-aged woman. As I swept my hands over her legs, I got a sense of "coldness" in her right knee. It was much colder than the left knee, the right hip, and the right ankle, which was surprisingly warm. So, I started working on the knee. She began to get restless. I worked a while longer and then re-assessed. It was still stone cold. Finally, I asked, "What's going on with your knee?" She replied, "There is nothing wrong with my knee. I had it replaced two years ago; it's my ankle that hurts!" This was a good reminder to check in and ask before leaping into treating. I sensed her knee was abnormal because it was artificial, but it wasn't causing any pain, and she didn't want it treated. I went back and worked on her ankle, and soon she said it was feeling much better. Initially, I had observed coolness at the knee and heat at the ankle, but I assessed the "problem" and need for intervention incorrectly because I had not checked in with the recipient. Lesson learned.

The way I was taught to do an assessment in Therapeutic Touch was to gently sweep my hands about two to six inches over the body's surface in short segments (six to eighteen inches at a time), starting with the head and ending with the feet. Over the torso, start with hands together in the midline and sweep outward, away from the center, keeping the hands moving, assessing both the front and back if possible. We usually did assessments in pairs with the recipient sitting on a short bench, stool, or backless chair, one of us standing behind the recipient and the other standing, kneeling, sitting, or squatting in front. This approach allows the healer to easily compare the right and left sides of the body, and doing the assessment with another person also helps double-check your observation and assessment with someone else. If you're alone, remember to assess both front and back of the body as feasible given the recipient's position. If I'm seeing someone who is reclining in bed or on an exam table, I often ask her to roll to one side so I can assess the back, too. Remember, you are not making a diagnosis; you are simply observing for differences in the right and left sides, front and back, higher and lower, and a general sense of flow, balance, order, and vitality.

Since I see a lot of patients who are reclining on exam tables or hospital beds and I don't usually have a partner doing assessments with me, I often incorporate a healer's assessment into a physician's physical exam. Just before or after listening to the heart and lungs, I often sweep gently over the front and back of the chest. Before listening to the belly, I place my hands gently over the abdomen and just see what I can sense with my hands. Before having the patient sit up for the neurologic exam, I lightly sweep my hands over both legs and then touch the knees and ankles.

As a pediatrician, I sometimes see toddlers who are afraid of being touched, and I've learned to start by holding their feet so they can see what I'm doing and that it isn't scary or painful. We may do the feet up to the knees and then the hands up to the elbows before listening to the heart and lungs, saving the head exam for last since so many small children dislike having their ears examined.

All of this detail is simply to say that we adapt our exam to meet the needs of the recipient in the moment. Having a routine helps us be systematic and not forget key parts of the assessment. It's also reassuring and predictable, so we can focus on our centering and grounding and observation rather than trying to think about what's next. Especially as you begin to do assessments, it is a good idea to develop a consistent routine. But don't let your routine become such a dogma that you are unable to adapt to the needs of the moment when the situation calls for it.

What Are You Likely to Sense When a Recipient Is Stressed?

Remember to look for the obvious. Every baby can tell when his mother is upset. What does she look like? She has a tense facial expression, the muscles of her shoulders and upper back are tense, she breathes a little faster and more shallowly than usual, her face may pale and wan, she may be sweating, and her voice is slightly higher pitched. She may cry or wring her hands. If her stress has turned to anger, she may be clenching her jaw, turning red with a throbbing vessel in the temple, speaking faster and more loudly, pointing and jabbing with her finger or pounding her fist.

As your sensitivity increases in your hands, you are likely to feel the tension in the shoulders even without touching them. You may feel an increased sense of heat over the temples, a spikiness or static over the head, and a sense of tightness over the chest. Healers who are very empathetic or kinesthetic may start to mirror and experience the same physical sensations and emotions that the recipient is experiencing. They may feel their own shoulders tighten or sense butterflies in their stomach, which tells them what the recipient is sensing in her body. This is one reason it is so important to be able to notice, observe, and determine where the feeling is coming from (you or the recipient) and return to your own sense of inner peace.

So, you are combining what you feel in your hands with what you observe with your eyes, ears, and other senses, including the sense inside your own body, while maintaining your connection with inner peace and goodwill.

After you finish your assessment, take a moment to check in with your partner (if you're working with one) to compare notes. If you're working alone, check in with the recipient. If you noticed coolness over the left side, note that the left side felt cooler than the right, and ask which side they would like to focus on.

Avoid telling a recipient that there is something "wrong" with a particular organ; not only might you be incorrect in your interpretation, but you may induce anxiety and start a series of unnecessary and unproductive laboratory and imaging tests. Healers do not make diagnoses. We are observing, assessing, interpreting, and addressing a sense of flow, balance, order, and vitality.

Step 3: Intervening to Restore Balance, Flow, Calm, and Relaxation

Remember to be clear about your goal. Once you have completed the assessment, return to your sense of inner peace and goodwill for the other person. You would like him to feel calm, confident, relaxed, balanced, and at ease. Imagine him feeling that way now. Make a plan.

There is an old saying in dermatology, "If it's dry, wet it. If it's wet, dry it. If it's inflamed, use steroids." In healing work, we use a similar principle: "If you sense heat, cool it. If you sense cool, warm it. If you sense prickly, smooth it. If you sense excess fullness, dissipate it. If you sense emptiness, fill it." Basically, try to restore a sense of balance, harmony, order, peace, and vitality.

You probably noticed during the warm-up exercises in the last chapter that some kinds of touch and sweeping motions were more calming and comforting than others. Standing behind a seated recipient and slowly sweeping from midline away to the sides of the head, from the forehead, across the temples, and over the ears is relaxing. Sweeping from the top of the head downward over the shoulders, and from the neck and shoulders down and outward across the back is more relaxing than sweeping upward or toward the midline. You can also stand at the seated recipient's side and sweep one hand down the face, neck, and chest in front while you stroke down the back of the head, neck, and back with the other. This sweeping or stroking motion can be off of the physical body (two to six inches above the body) or very lightly touching. Trust your intuition, and verify with the recipient what is comfortable. You may think of a metaphor of using a large, wide-tooth comb and gently untangling hair. Or you may think of it as petting a friendly dog or cat, a little off of the body.

Don't be afraid to ask for feedback from the recipient. Some people don't like anyone moving something in front of their eyes. Some are very sensitive to movement or touch over their throat. Women often don't like a stranger's hands too close to their breasts. Pay attention to body language, and when in doubt, ask.

If the recipient is reclining on his back, I usually make gentle sweeps from the forehead to the bed or table (stand at the head of the bed/table). Then I move around to his side and sweep from the top of the chest down over the abdomen, timing sweeps to coincide with slow, deep breaths, breathing in as I bring my hands back to a starting position, and breathing out as I sweep my hands downward and outward.

A healing intervention for stress doesn't usually require much attention to the arms and hands or lower belly, but many people find it comforting to have their wrists and hands held briefly. Those who are so stressed that they feel nauseous may be comforted by slow downward strokes over their belly, with a sense of soothing downward motion, off the body. Continue down the hips, thighs, legs, and feet. You can repeat the sweeping movements several times over any areas that feel like they need a little extra attention; this is often the case over the shoulders and upper back in someone who is stressed. Keep the hands moving until you get to the feet. I often spend time holding a person's feet to give her a tactile sense of being grounded—in the sense of being connected to someone else or to the earth. Particularly for someone whose stress has led to hyperventilation and dizziness, it can be helpful to hold his feet and encourage him to imagine he can take slow, deep breaths through the soles of his feet, breathing out through the feet into the ground.

Step 4: Re-assessment

When you've finished addressing whatever sense of imbalance you detected, or restoring a sense of flow or vitality, it is helpful to go back and re-assess the whole person. Sometimes you will detect an additional area that may benefit from some attention. Sometimes you will notice you want to do a full-body treatment to pull everything together after focusing on a smaller area. If you are a health professional, this is an opportunity to re-assess vital signs, pain, and other measures routinely collected and recorded in a clinical setting.

How Long Does a Session Last?

This question is a little like asking how long does a meal last or how much food you should eat. You should eat until you are slightly less than full—your body will tell you when. A typical healing session lasts about twenty minutes; sessions take less time for children and those who are weak or debilitated. For someone who is basically strong and filled with vitality (as when trading treatments with another healer), you can go longer if you both enjoy the process. Trust your intuition, and when in doubt, ask.

How Do You End a Session?

I usually end a session by bringing my hands back to rest on the recipient's shoulders, taking a couple of deep, slow breaths, and thanking the recipient. At times I will end a session holding the recipient's feet. If you are working with another healer, one of you can hold the feet while the other holds the shoulders. Remind the recipient that when she's ready, she can open her eyes, or rest with eyes closed a few minutes longer.

I thank the patient and ask if there's anything else that would like additional attention right now. If not, I ask how she's doing, ask about stress or relaxation on the zero-to-ten scale, and explain that it's normal to feel relaxed and sleepy for a while after a session. On the other hand, some people feel energized and hungry. Some people don't feel any different. That's okay, too, and it doesn't mean the session hasn't been worthwhile. If you have been able to maintain a sense of being centered and grounded while extending goodwill, kindness, and peacefulness to the recipient, it's been worthwhile. Remember to wash your hands and make some notes in the official health record or your practice journal.

Offer to let the recipient rest for several minutes after a session. Usually recipients become very relaxed, and it's worthwhile to let them experience that deep relaxation a bit longer. In our workshops, we often let recipients rest for fifteen to thirty minutes after a treatment, taking a mini-nap and soaking it all in. This is usually easier to do in a workshop or hospital room than in a clinic room that needs to be cleaned quickly for the next patient. If you're working in a clinic space with high turnover rates, encourage the recipient to just rest in the waiting room for a few minutes before rushing home. If you are working in a hospice or home setting, you can just let the recipient rest where she is.

Anything Else?

We have covered the basics. Yet, there are many variations on these simple themes. Some healers use calm, relaxing music during a session, while others prefer the power of silence. Some use relaxing aromatherapy like lavender or chamomile, while others prefer a scent-free environment.

For older children and adults who can use their imagination to help the healing process, I often ask them to help me by taking *slow, deep breaths* with me. I ask them to put one or both hands on their belly so they can feel it rise as they breathe in and fall as they breathe out. As they take their first breath in, I breathe with them, matching their pace for several breaths, reassuring them that they are doing very well with this breathing. Then I slow down my breathing just a little. If you have established a shared rhythm, the recipient will usually slow down with you, and you can reassure them that it is okay to slow down and relax. Keep observing, and from time to time, provide positive reinforcement ("nice job," "nice, slow breaths," "good, relaxing breathing," etc.).

As you do your work, you may notice the recipient's leg twitch or other muscles jerk. This is a sign that they are starting to relax. You can comment on that softly, "That twitch is a sign that your muscles are relaxing. Good job."

As the recipient relaxes with deep breathing, you may also help guide their imagination to a time and place they felt safe and relaxed, a place in nature, a time on vacation, or it might be an imaginary place they've seen in a movie or read about in a book. They don't need to tell you about it, but they can imagine it vividly—the colors, the light, who and what was there, the sounds, the aromas, the feeling of sunlight and a breeze on the skin. Vividly imagining being in a safe, peaceful place actually prompts our bodies to react as if we were there, helping us relax.

An overhead page beckoned me "stat" to the post-operative recovery area. When I arrived, I found an anesthesiologist and nurse hovering over 15-year-old Jane's bedside. I had seen Jane the month before when she was hospitalized for recurrent pneumonia; Therapeutic Touch and guided imagery helped her feel better. Now she was heavily sedated following a procedure, and the team had called me because her coughing was so severe that she required strong sedation and a breathing tube to keep her oxygen levels up. Her mother insisted that they call me to offer a healing session in addition to the outstanding medical care she was already receiving. So, I did what had worked for her before. In a calm, friendly, relaxed, curious way, I asked her to imagine herself in her favorite place, which I knew from the month earlier was red convertible, riding down the California coastal highway with her mom; we vividly evoked that memory—the sights, the sounds, the smell of the ocean, the feeling of the wind in her face. At the same time, my hands made slow, sweeping, downward movements over her chest and belly to reinforce the feeling of peaceful relaxation. Gradually the nurse reduced the sedative medicine, and within ten minutes, Jane's breathing tube was out and she was breathing easily without coughing. Integrative health care combines the best of conventional care and healing strategies, such as guided imagery.

What about Colors?

As you offer healing to the recipient, as you gently hold his shoulders and make sweeps over his body (or hold your hands still over his heart, hands, or feet), you may want to use *your* imagination, too. Many healers imagine they are drawing on Universal Healing Energy in the form of clear or white light from the heavens pouring down through their heads, into the heart, and out through their hands into the recipient. This imagery reinforces the notion that the healer is not using up her own energy, but simply serving as a channel or vehicle, which helps avoid the problems of pride and arrogance. It also helps us stay energized and avoids depleting our own personal energy stores.

In addition to clear or white light, a deep, royal blue is often a very soothing color that can be imagined as flowing through the healer's hands into the recipient. Imagine the healing, comforting light flowing into you as you breathe in and flowing out through your hands as you breathe out. It circulates just where it needs to go, and any excess light or energy can easily flow out through the breath or

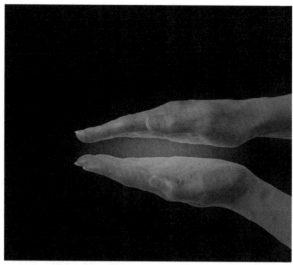

© Nikki Zalewski – Fotolia.com

down through the feet into the earth. The important thing is not the color per se but the feeling it generates in the healer because her mental and emotional state of well-being, safety, relaxation, vitality, order, and strength impacts the recipient.

Remember, of the five steps in healing, steps 1, 2, and 5 are most important. Relax and enjoy the process. Wash your hands.

1. Center on the stillness, peace, wisdom, compassion, and harmony within that connects you with your deepest self and something greater than yourself. Maintain that center throughout all other steps. Maintain your grounding in your intention to extend peace and goodwill to the recipient.

2. Observe the recipient using your eyes, ears, and hands with an open, non-judgmental, kind, caring awareness. When in doubt, ask. After you assess, form an intention and make a plan.

3. Use your hands either gently on or slightly off the body, either still or moving, to help restore a sense of balance, relaxation, calm, confidence, and an easy flow throughout the body. Consider asking the recipient to assist by using his breathing and imagination. Consider using your imagination, too.

4. Re-assess and address anything that seems to need extra attention.

5. When you feel finished, maintain a curious, accepting, non-judgmental non-attachment to results. Return again to your inner sense of peace and compassion. Tell the recipient softly that you are finished, thank him, and ask how he is feeling and if any additional treatment is desired. Wash your hands. Keep notes in the health record or your journal.

Remember to let the healing session flow easily. Trying too hard reflects a lack of confidence and stress. The more you can relax and trust the process, the more easily the recipient can relax and feel calm and confident.

"Try not to try too hard. It's just a lovely ride."
—JAMES TAYLOR, "SECRET O' LIFE"

Chronic stress is draining. After a long period of illness, pain, or stress, a person may feel deeply fatigued. In these situations, your goal may be to restore a sense of calm, vitality, and energy. That's what the next chapter is all about.

CHAPTER 13

Energizing and Building Vitality

ALTHOUGH THE MAJORITY of patients seek help for stress or pain, a substantial number have been sick for so long that they have become fatigued. For anyone who is frail or fatigued, use brief sessions. Just as a person who is starving can become ill by eating too much too quickly, a person who is very fatigued and debilitated can become worse by having an excessively lengthy or intense session. Be gentle, and err on the side of under- rather than over-treatment.

Always start with these two steps:

1. Centering and grounding yourself, being clear about your intention. Wash your hands and prepare yourself, the recipient, others present, and the environment for a healing interaction.
2. Assess the recipient and the situation before plunging ahead. Observe carefully, and ask the person what is going on and what her goals are for the session.

As you reflect on the assessment and plan your strategy, remember the basics: "If it's warm, cool it. If it's cool, warm it. If it's full, move it. If it's depleted, fill it." Your overall goal is to restore a sense of balance, vitality, order, comfort, and peace.

Also recall that even when it appears still and static, the healthy human body is constantly in motion. The heart is pumping about once a second; the brain waves are going four to fifteen cycles per second; the lungs are breathing in and out ten to twenty times a minute; the intestinal tract is contracting and moving the contents along about three times a minute; and, even the endocrine glands are creating and releasing hormones in their own rhythms throughout the day. So, maintain a sense of harmonious rhythm and dynamic flow in your actions.

If your assessment reveals areas that feel hot or full, move your hands over them from above to below, center to periphery, extending imagery of cooling or moving the heat out, releasing it into the earth.

For example, if someone has rheumatoid arthritis and feels very tired, you may want to help her feel more energetic, but you don't want to make the pain worse. So, if you sense a heat or fullness over the hands, cool and move that out by sweeping from the shoulders down to the fingertips and beyond before starting to help build vitality.

Similarly, if someone has a tumor or serious infection like pneumonia, you will want to give that area some specific attention before helping build vitality.

For the sake of simplicity, let's just say we are going to work with someone who is chronically fatigued and doesn't have any other specific concern—no arthritis, cancer, high blood pressure, diabetes, infections—just fatigue. When you do your assessment, you don't notice any particular areas of heat, tingling, or fullness, just a general sense of fatigue and low vitality.

What are you likely to notice when you assess someone who is fatigued? Her movements are minimal and slow. The head may hang, the shoulders may droop, the speech is slow, and the voice sounds quiet and flat. The skin may be pale or white. In your own body, if you are kinesthetic, you may feel slower, colder, and more tired. When you pass your hands over her body, you might notice that you need to get much closer than usual to feel the normal sense of heat or vitality.

General Approach to Balancing and Re-vitalizing: The Foot Bone Connects to the Anklebone

Remember the song "The Foot Bone's Connected to the Anklebone"? That's how I think of this strategy to restore a sense of vitality.

I'm going to assume you've already washed your hands,

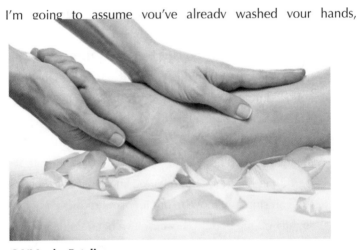

© VI Levi – Fotolia.com

centered, grounded, and completed your assessment (steps 1 and 2 above), and planned to help restore a sense of balance and vitality. I'm also going to assume the recipient is reclining on her back and your dominant hand is your right hand, so you are standing to the

KATHI J. KEMPER, M.D., M.P.H.

right of the recipient (if your dominant hand is left, by now you are used to translating directions to the opposite side).

1. Start with the recipient's right foot. Put the palm of your right hand on the sole of the recipient's right foot[153], and the palm of your left hand over the top of the foot. Hold them there as you engage your imagination. Imagine that as you breathe in, you are drawing energy from Mother Earth. This is gentle, but powerful, nurturing, healing, restorative energy that flows upward through your legs, into your heart, and as you breathe out, it flows down your arms, through your right hand, through the recipient's foot, filling it up. Whatever is not needed is or is excess flows through into your left hand, and from there, wherever it needs to go. For the first few breaths, you might not feel anything in your left hand, but as you continue, you will start to feel the sense of connection and flow into your left hand. As this happens, you might also notice that the recipient's foot starts to feel warmer[154] between your hands. As I begin, I usually prepare the recipient, asking her to tell me when she starts to feel warmth in her foot, and to let me know if it ever gets too hot so I can stop and move to another spot or move my hands slightly off the body[155]. Because I've been doing this kind of thing longer than most recipients have received healing

---

153 If you enjoyed studying Chinese meridians, put your palm over the spot known as Kidney 1.
154 Or it might feel tingling or full or "done." Pay attention to the signal that something is changing; the signal may be different for you than it is for me.
155 No one has ever told me it's gotten too hot, but giving the recipient a sense of control and the expectation that something powerful is about to happen are very helpful suggestions.

sessions, I usually feel the connection between my hands a moment or two before the recipient, but sometimes she feels it first. When I have a solid sense of connection, I move on. If you linger too long, you may notice that restlessness develops in you or the recipient.

2. Keep the right hand on the sole of the foot, and move the left hand to the ankle. This slightly increases the distance between the hands. Maintain the imagery of drawing healing, nurturing vitality up from Mother Earth as you breathe in, just as a tree draws nutrients up its roots. As you breathe out, let it flow from your heart through the right hand, along the recipient's foot bones, into the anklebones, and out into your left hand. When you feel a solid sense of connection between your hands, it's time to move to the next step.

3. Next, move your left hand up to the kneecap and repeat the process. This time that connection travels all the way up the shinbone, into your left hand, filling the recipient's lower leg from the inside out. When you feel the sense of connection between your hands, move the left hand up to the hip bone or the front of the pelvic bone and repeat.

4. It's important for the foot-bone-to-anklebone exercise to use your imagination to "run the energy" upward through the bones. While we generally send the soothing, stress-reducing message sweeping downward along the outside of the body, relaxing skin, connective tissue, and muscle, we extend revitalizing energy upward along the very center of the bones, from the bottom to the top, from the inside out.

5. After you've finished the right leg from the bottom of the foot up to the hip, move your right hand to the sole of the left foot and repeat the process up the entire left leg.

6. There is a learning process with this work, and many times you will feel the flow faster on one side than the other side as you get used to working. You may not. If the person is debilitated or for some reason resisting the treatment (despite the request for it), the process may seem sluggish. If your intuition tells you to move on, move on, even if you don't feel a strong sense of connection or flow between your hands. Do pause for at least two or three breaths at every joint to establish an orderly sense of connection, balance, and flow.

7. When you've finished working your way up the legs, it's time for the trunk. I generally place my right hand over the lower belly between the hip bones and just above the pubic bone, and my left hand just slightly farther up the belly. When that connection seems solid, I move the left hand up to the solar plexus. On a smaller person, I may able to cover the entire upper belly with my hand, but on a larger person, I will repeat the process over the upper left side and then the upper right side of the upper belly, just under the ribs.

8. If you are feeling a strong sense of connection each time, leave the right hand over the lower belly. If the connection seems weak, particularly when your hands are farther apart, move the right hand up to solar plexus as you move the left hand over the middle of the chest, palm over the sternum. Keep up your breathing, slow, steady, and rhythmic. Be aware of the subtle movements of the recipient that indicate their degree of relaxation or tension. For teenage girls and adult women, I usually ask if it's okay to touch the middle of their chest. If they feel uncomfortable with that,

I hold the left hand one to three inches over the body, not touching it.

9. As you move from the chest upward toward the throat, again be aware that many people do not like having their throat touched. You can either hold your hand above the throat, or place your left hand on the collarbone on the left and right sides for two separate connections. When you've finished, move your left hand to the right shoulder.

10. With your left hand on the right shoulder, place your right palm against the recipient's right palm. If their hand is down and this seems awkward, just place the palm of your right hand over the back of the recipient's right hand. Continue breathing. When you're ready, move your right hand up to the inside of the recipient's right elbow. When you've established a nice sense of connection along the right arm, move your left hand to the recipient's left shoulder.

11. With your left hand on the recipient's left shoulder, touch or hold the recipient's left hand with your right hand and repeat the process. If the recipient is a very big person and it's uncomfortable for you to reach, you can walk around the table or bed and switch hands on the left side.

12. After completing both arms, move the right hand either to the place where the collarbones meet, the middle of the chest, or the solar plexus, whatever seems best to you, and the left hand over the top of the head. I usually have my left hand off the top of the body at this point and connect here only briefly. Having the hands still over the head can be uncomfortable for many recipients, so I don't linger long here without moving.

13. If the recipient is not snoring or otherwise obviously deeply

relaxed, I ask if there's any place that would like to have a stronger sense of connection, and I repeat that connection for her. Usually, however, they feel nice and comfortable, and I repeat the assessment from head to toe with slow, sweeping motions about two to six inches over the body to check for any areas that seem like they would benefit from some brief attention. Typically, you will notice that the skin has turned from pale to slightly pink and from dry to moist, the breathing is slower and steadier, things seem more balanced, and you can feel the recipient's vitality a bit farther away from the body than you did with the initial assessment.

14. Often after completing the foot-bone-to-anklebone process, I reverse the flow, doing a few long, gentle sweeps from head to toe, to re-assess the entire person and encourage a state of balanced, gentle flow.

15. Finish by holding the recipient's shoulders or feet and letting them know you are done. Ask how they are feeling on the 0 to 10 scale, how they experienced the session, and ask for feedback so you can properly document in your treatment journal or the recipient's health record. Wash your hands. Remember, the outcome of the treatment is not up to you. Release the results. Maintain compassionate, kind curiosity about what unfolds.

People who are fatigued also usually have had trouble sleeping. Either they can't fall asleep, or they wake up and can't fall asleep again, or they have restless sleep or awaken without feeling refreshed. So, don't be surprised if your intervention doesn't make the recipient leap off the table, but instead sends her for a nap.

One day I was treating a teenage boy whose father had driven him from another state to see me for his chronic fatigue and insomnia. He had mono the previous fall and recovered for a few weeks only to develop influenza in the winter. Even though he'd recovered from the pneumonia, his energy had never come back, and he was missing a lot of school, was unable to sleep at night, and was unable to keep his eyes open in class. After the "foot-bone-to-anklebone" treatment, the son rested a few minutes while I chatted with his dad. I cautioned him that different people respond differently, and that even if his son felt fantastic afterward, he should enjoy the feeling and not try to run a marathon or play an intense game of one-on-one basketball that day. His father called me from their hotel the next morning to tell me how the afternoon had gone. "He was unbelievable as we left the clinic," he reported. "He was jumping up trying to touch the ceiling beams in the parking garage and laughing all the way to the car; he told me he was starving for a burger, and he finished the whole thing. We got back to the hotel and he slept for four hours straight without stirring. He got up for dinner, watched a game with me on TV, went to bed at ten p.m., and slept through solidly till seven a.m. today. I feel like I've got my boy back! Thank you!" I cautioned him that he still needed to take it slow, and we went over some other medical issues (his vitamin D was low and needed to be restored, as well). Three months later, he came back for a follow-up visit and reported that although he'd had some ups and downs, he had turned the corner, was finishing the semester on time, was sleeping well, and was back to sports.

Not every recipient will respond as quickly and completely as

KATHI J. KEMPER, M.D., M.P.H.

this teenage boy. Someone who is basically healthy generally recovers more quickly than someone who has been chronically fatigued for years. Someone with no other health problems generally responds more quickly and completely than someone with a serious chronic condition like cancer, AIDS, or multiple sclerosis. On the other hand, I've seen dramatic improvements in children with serious conditions, too. Keep your mind open, and maintain a sense of compassionate curiosity about the process, dedicated to doing your part, but remaining unattached to the outcome. Remember the difference between healing and curing, and do not think of healing work as a replacement for conventional medical care.

As Part of a More Targeted Strategy

The "foot-bone-to-anklebone" technique is a useful general strategy for fatigue, particularly for those who've had insomnia as well as fatigue. Fatigue and a sense of low vitality or energy can also accompany acute illnesses. Remember the last time you had bad cold or the flu? You probably just wanted to crawl under the covers until the whole thing was over. That's the wisdom of the body to use its precious life force or energy for healing rather than tackling work or chores.

If your assessment reveals localized areas of fullness, heat, cool, buzzing, or something else that feels as if it needs the opposite, do give those areas the attention they need. If I see someone with fullness and heat over the chest (e.g., someone with pneumonia or bronchitis), I try to clear and cool the chest before I do the "foot bone to anklebone." Similarly, for other acute situations like sinus infections, colds, or even sprained ankles, first clear, balance, and restore flow if possible where it is needed. After you tend to the local areas that need it, you may no longer need to do the full-body treatment. Or you can use the full-body treatment as a complement to a focal strategy. Follow your intuition.

Other Tools for Helping Restore Vitality

You may have noticed in the "foot-bone-to-anklebone" strategy that I suggested involving the recipient in letting you know when she felt the connection. This not only sets the expectation that she will experience something, but it also empowers her as part of the treatment. For those who are able, consider inviting them to participate in other ways, too.

1. Recipients can use their imagination to bolster the effects of the treatment by imagining life force energy or vitality or Mother Earth's healing energy flowing into their feet and up their bones. They may see this as colors, hear it as music, or feel it like water or the warmth of a cozy fire.

2. Healers can use their imaginations, too. What colors evoke a sense of comfortable vitality for you? Are they warm, autumnal colors like gold and green, or pastels like baby blue, lavender, or pink? What about music? Do you prefer to dwell on a rousing march, an inspiring hymn, a popular dance number, a movie theme by John Williams? Engage your senses on as many levels as possible. When we vividly experience the sense of vitality, enthusiasm, balance, harmony, order, and well-being, we unconsciously, non-verbally communicate it with others, including others in the room. There is no one right answer to what fills you with a sense of vigor, and it's likely to be somewhat unique for each person. The important thing is to impart that sense of

strength and vitality to the recipient through your intention, your presence, and your caring touch.

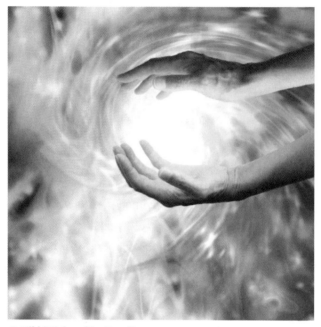

© **Nikki Zalewski – Fotolia.com**

Now that we've covered strategies to address stress and fatigue, let's experience and practice tools to offer comfort and ease to someone who has a painful condition. That's what the next chapter is about.

CHAPTER 14

Offering Comfort and Reducing Pain

ASIDE FROM UTTERING A FEW selected heartfelt words, what's the first thing you do when you bump your head? Grab your head. Hit your finger with a hammer? Grab your finger. Hit your shin on the coffee table? Grab your leg. When we're hurt, the first thing most of us do is grab that part that hurts. Holding the hurt is natural.

As a healer, you will be asked to help those who are in pain. And you will be expected to touch or hold the painful part. First, do no harm. Sometimes you can't touch the hurt directly. For burns, cuts, scrapes, and skin infections, please do not directly touch the wound. Avoid spreading infections.

Before any session, whether you touch or not, wash your hands. And if someone doesn't want to be touched, don't.

Plenty of data support the helpfulness of techniques used in Therapeutic Touch, Healing Touch, and Reiki to ease pain[156]. So does personal experience.

---

156 Henneghan A.M. and Schnyer R.N., "Biofield therapies for symptom management in palliative and end-of-life care," *American Journal of Hospice and Palliative Care* (November 20, 2013). Lu D.F., Hart L.K., Lutgendorf S.K., and Perkhounkova Y., "The effect of healing touch on the pain and mobility of persons with osteoarthritis: a feasibility study," *Geriatr Nurs* 34, no. 4 (2013): 314–22. Anderson J.G. and Taylor A.G., "Biofield therapies and cancer pain, *Clin J Oncol Nurs* 16, no. 1 (2012): 43–8. Monroe C.M., "The effects of therapeutic touch on pain," *J Holist Nurs*, 2009; 27(2): 85–92. Kemper KJ, Kelly EA. Treating children with therapeutic and healing touch. *Pediatr Ann* 33, no. 4 (2004): 248–52. Wardell D.W., Decker S.A., Engebretson J.C., "Healing touch for older adults with persistent pain," *Holistic Nurse Practitioner* 26, no. 4 (2012): 194–202.

My introduction to Therapeutic Touch came in 1985 when I developed a migraine headache while visiting my friend, Helen. Helen invited me to the kitchen, where she offered to give me something that would help. I sat on a kitchen stool, my head in my hands, waiting for her to open a bottle of pain pills. Instead, she stepped behind me and started waving her hands over my head. I wondered, "Where is the pain medicine?" But it was her house. I was a guest, and I didn't want to insult her, so I sat there wondering what was going on and how soon I could reasonably go home, take some ibuprofen, and rest in the dark. Her hands felt like static electricity was building up over my head as she continued to stroke the air around my head. Weird. But then I noticed something really strange. My headache was going away. Literally moment by moment, the intensity decreased. I had never experienced anything like it before. "What are you doing?" I demanded to know. "Therapeutic Touch," she responded. "Well, I need to learn how to do that," I said. "If I have a patient with a headache in the hospital, the nurse notifies me to come do an evaluation, I make a diagnosis, order the medicine; the order goes to the pharmacy; the medication is dispensed; the nurse takes it to the patient; the patient takes the medicine; and thirty to forty minutes later, the patient starts to feel better. This whole process means that hospitalized headache patients wait at least an hour for relief, but THIS offers relief in minutes, requires only one person, and is very safe. How can I learn to do that?" Helen told me about the training programs led by Dora Kunz and Dolores Krieger, RN, Ph.D. And a few years later, I had the opportunity to start studying with them myself.

Here are a few of those helpful techniques. Some of them were learned from Dora and Dolores, and a few I've learned along the way. One of the first techniques I learned in Therapeutic Touch was to help with headache pain with smoothing motions like those Helen had used with me.

1. Smooth the Suffering

Before using any technique to help promote a greater sense of ease and comfort, remember the basics: Wash your hands. Ask the recipient to sit or recline in a comfortable, supported position. Check to make sure lighting, sounds, music, fragrances, temperature, pillows, blankets, people present, and so forth are to the recipient's liking as much as possible. If appropriate, hang a "do not disturb" sign on the door.

a. Focus on your own center of peace and calm, and maintain your grounding in your positive intention toward the recipient achieving an optimal state of well-being.

b. Do an assessment using careful, compassionate, non-judgmental observation. Avoid the temptation of impulsively jumping in to work at the obvious site of pain. For example, headache pain may actually come from grinding the jaw, stuffy sinuses, or tight shoulder muscles. Knee pain may actually come from a problem with the hip or ankle, or even the back. Make a plan. Some people start by soothing the stress (which is almost always present for people in pain; see Chapter 12). Some start by increasing the vitality of the whole person (often the case if someone has become debilitated with chronic pain; see Chapter 13), and then

225

focus on the pain. For more recent pain in which the sufferer is generally calm, treatment usually starts with the most painful site and then expands to the whole person. Any of these approaches or combinations can work. Remember, you can ask the recipient what he would prefer. Just make sure you make a plan that includes working with the part that hurts, as well as the whole person, and includes an assessment afterward. Let's say that you plan to start with the part that hurts, for example, a headache.[157]

c. Involve the recipient. As part of your assessment, you will probably ask how uncomfortable the pain is on a 0 to 10 scale in which 0 means completely comfortable (no pain) and 10 means severe discomfort or pain. Ask the recipient how low they would like their number to go with this treatment (their comfort goal). Asking at the beginning helps establish the sense that improvement is possible, and positive expectations are linked to better outcomes.

d. For headaches, we typically stand or sit behind the recipient, either behind his chair or at the head of the bed. Starting with forehead, sweep the hands gently about two to six inches off the body toward the back of the head. Maintain a sense that you are *smoothing away* the headache as you repeat this sweeping motion. I generally start with the middle of the forehead and sweep across the sides and down the middle of the back of the head. I gradually cover the whole head, starting from the front to the back of the head, and then down over the shoulders and upper back. Be sure to include the eyes, sinuses, and

---

157 Krieger D., *The Personal Practice of Therapeutic Touch*, (Santa Fe: Bear and Company, 1993), 158–9.

jaw. Smoothing motions at a steady, rhythmic, calm pace help promote a sense of calm and ease. Consider timing your hand motions with your breath to create an overall sense of harmony and order.

Consider using your imagination. Imagine the headache as tangled hair and your hands as a comb with widely spaced teeth gradually loosening and straightening those tangles. Or imagine the headache like sharp spikes sticking up out of the head, gradually worn down by repeated smoothing strokes. Or imagine the headache as heat waves being cooled with soothing watery streams from your hands. If you are more auditory, you might hear jarring or uncomfortable sounds that you imagine replacing with soothing tones. If you are more kinesthetic, you might imagine tense, tight muscles gradually relaxing. The specific image matters less than the general mental and emotional sense of restoring calm order, ease, and comfort.

Be patient. It often takes three to five minutes for the recipient to begin to relax and feel more comfortable.

Continue to involve the recipient. Ask him to tell you when the number for their discomfort (from 0 to 10) falls one number lower than the starting number (or 0.1 or 0.5 for those whose pain has been stuck at one level for a long time). When you reach that number, ask when the next lower number is attained[158]. This sets an attitude of positive expectation, or at least neutral curiosity. Remind the recipient that you can stop or change what you're doing at any time if he would like something different or more of something that was par-

---

158 Note that asking the recipient to participate is something I've started doing after I trained with Dora and Dolores. I treat children, and they don't like sitting still for long without doing something. When I ask them to become involved by telling me when they reach the next number lower, they become expectant and curious, and this open-minded attention is just what we want.

ticularly helpful. This helps empower the recipient as a co-participant in the healing process.

If you get stuck at a number higher than your goal, switch to a total-body focus. After doing a total-body treatment (either sweeping along the entire body to help decrease stress or doing the foot-bone-to-anklebone technique described in earlier chapters), return to the primary site of discomfort. Sometimes just improving the overall sense of flow, balance, and vitality will allow the next phase of improvement to unfold more easily.

a. Re-assess the whole person. Focus on any other areas that need some extra attention.
b. I generally close by gently holding the recipient's feet or shoulders, letting him know quietly that he can rest here a while, and when he's ready, gently stretch fingers and toes, hands and feet, come back to an awareness of the room, and open his eyes. Wash your hands and jot down your own notes about the session while the recipient rests. Remember, you do your best, and the healing is in the hands of the recipient. Maintain your sense of inner peace (centering), goodwill (grounding), and non-attachment. Ask for feedback so you can learn and continue to improve. If the comfort level is better, remind the recipient how he was able to use that time and experience to achieve his goal. Do not claim credit for improvements. The person who improves (the recipient) is the true healer.

Smoothing the suffering is the most common healing strategy we use to help with pain, whether the pain is from a headache or a sprained ankle or a tummy ache.

Smoothing Suffering Variation 1:

For recipients who have migraine headaches, other symptoms often include nausea and sensitivity to light and sound, as well as throbbing head pain. In these situations, some recipients feel better with hands still (one over the forehead and one over the nape of the neck). You may then create a sense of downward flow and connection by sweeping downward over the chest and belly toward the feet (hands moving). Or you can hold the dominant hand over the back of the neck and the non-dominant hand over the belly; then shift the hands down so the dominant hand is on the belly and the non-dominant hand is on the knees, feet, or ground. Either way, you maintain a sense of moving the discomfort downward and out of the body into the ground.

Smoothing Suffering Variation 2:

"Point Out" the Pain: This technique is specific for headaches and other pain in the face, head, and upper body. It is a non-needle acupuncture technique. As part of an overall treatment for pain, consider taking a moment or two to focus on the acupoints on the backs of both hands in the middle of the muscle between the bones leading to the thumb and pointer finger[159]. Here are two ways to work on those paired points (one at a time): a) acupressure: press on the acupoints with your thumb or pointer finger (it's okay to sandwich the point between thumb and pointer finger[160]; or b) imagine a stimulating energy flowing from the tips of your thumb, pointer, and long finger (held

---

159 In Chinese medicine, these points are called Large Intestine 4 (the fourth point on the large intestine meridian) or "hegu."
160 I have used this technique on myself when I developed a headache while driving at the end of the day and the sun was at a low angle, glaring directly into my eyes. My headache clears within five minutes of pressure to the hegu points.

lightly together as if you're holding a very thin pen) focused on the acupoint in small clockwise circles.

Smoothing Suffering Variation 3:

Hands to the Head: Regardless of the location or cause of the pain, I often sense heat over the top left side of the head, a bit above and in front of the ear, and as I work on soothing and cooling that heat, both on the head and the areas where the recipient experiences pain, his pain level drops. This is also where I sense their pain level. Over the years of working with children, some of whom cannot readily assign a number to pain, I've found this location a good "pain thermometer." Older patients are often astonished when I correctly guess their pain level simply from observing them closely, with attention to the sensation of heat over the left side of their head. I have not read about this elsewhere or heard it from any of my teachers. This is my personal experience. Your experience may be different. Please let me know what YOU observe as you help people in pain. You may find that you are more sensitive to other visual or auditory cues or different physical sensations in your hands or your own body.

2. Drain the Pain

Strategy 1 called for soothing the pain, which is usually done with soothing sweeps slightly off of the skin. A variation relies on the same kind of hand movements focused over the left side of the head. Strategy 2, Drain the Pain, involves hands that are still, with one hand actually touching the body. When I first learned about it from a Healing Touch-trained nurse, Mary Jane Ott, in Boston, I was dubious. But as I witnessed her patients relax and grow more comfortable as she did it, I decided to give it a try.

a. As with all healing strategies, begin by taking a conscious breath, focusing on being centered and grounded; wash your hands; make sure the recipient is comfortable; and address the things you can in the environment (temperature, sound/music, light level, pillows or blankets, privacy)

b. Observe and assess. Ask where the pain[161] or discomfort is worst, ask how severe it is on the 0 to 10 scale, and ask if it's okay to touch that area gently to ease the pain. Reassure the recipient that you can back off or touch the air over the area if it hurts too much to touch it directly, but that most people find this strangely soothing.

c. Place one hand over the part that hurts. You have a choice about the other hand: i) let it hang in the air pointing toward the ground; ii) touch the ground directly; iii) touch a bedrail or other piece of furniture that touches the ground. The point is to create the sense of a circuit from the painful part of the recipient's body to the ground.

Use your imagination in conjunction with your breathing. Remember, you are safe, peaceful, and comfortable, and you are not taking on anyone else's pain. As you breathe in, imagine that your hand that is touching the recipient is drawing his pain out of his body, up into your hand, up your arm, into your heart, down the other arm, and as you breathe out, the pain is draining down your other hand

---

161 Some pain treatment specialists avoid using the term "pain" when talking with patients. Instead, they call it "discomfort" and frame the goal in terms of increasing comfort rather than decreasing pain. There are sound psychological reasons for focusing on the positive goal of comfort, but there are times when it's more expedient to call a spade a spade and just call it pain and pain relief. Either way, even young children understand the concept of zero being no pain (good) and ten being terrible pain (bad). Whenever possible, be aware of and use the terms used by the recipient; this promotes a sense of empathetic understanding. For recipients, feeling understood is therapeutic in itself.

and into the ground. Your breath is like a pump, pumping the pain out of his body, through your heart, and draining it down into the earth. The pain doesn't stop anywhere in your body. Your hands, arms, and heart are simply acting as conduits. Your intention and your breath are the pumps pulling the pain out and allowing it to drain away into the earth. None of it sticks to you. Just as the earth welcomes compost and uses it to nurture living plants, the earth knows what to do to turn this pain into something nurturing. The pain that drains into the earth will not hurt the earth or anyone else.

Just as it often takes a water pump a few minutes of pumping before water starts to flow, you may notice that it seems to take a few deep breaths before the pain starts draining[162]. Be patient. Give it at least ten good pumping, draining breaths before you shift to another strategy.

When you feel finished with draining the pain, you probably are. Check with the recipient about his pain/comfort level at this point.

At this point, some people turn to the rest of body, while others turn to part 2 of the focus on this particular painful area. Part 2 involves filling the now emptied area with a sense of comfort and well-being. For part 2, move the "outflow" or "drainage" hand that had been on the ground onto the painful part, and move the hand that had been on the painful part upward into a position of receptivity. You can hold it up in the air, or palm up on your lap, or some other position that signifies to you that your hand is receiving a universal healing balm. Again, using your breath as a pump, breathe in the universal healing balm through the receiving hand, down the arm,

162 It may feel more like it's breaking up, softening, or shifting to a different sensation, or that it's being pulled out. Pay attention to your own experience, and don't be afraid to ask the recipient how things are shifting for him.

into your heart, and out into the area that had been painful, filling it up with a stream of beautiful, comforting healing. Continue until it feels nice and just right.

    a. Consider a series of head-to-toe sweeps to encourage a sense of comfortable flow. Re-assess, addressing any other areas that need attention.

    b. Close, as usual, by gently holding the recipient's shoulders or feet, inviting him to rest and encouraging his hands and feet to move and eyes to open if they've been closed. While the recipient rests, wash your hands, jot your notes, and ask for feedback so you can continue to improve. Take a few deep breaths to release attachment to results and re-focus on your sense of peace and compassion.

Variations on Draining the Pain

As with all techniques, there are variations that you might find interesting or useful for you or a recipient.

Drain the Pain Variation 1

In this transformational, compassionate healing meditation practice, at the third step, imagine there is a beautiful crystal in the area of your heart. (Don't worry, it's an imaginary crystal, and it doesn't displace your actual heart, lungs, or other organs.) This crystal has the power of transformation. Like the earth, it can take in waste and transform it into life-giving nutrients. But in this case, instead of transforming compost into plant food, this beautiful, heart-centered crystal can take pain and transform it into soothing, comforting, healing beams

KATHI J. KEMPER, M.D., M.P.H.

of beautiful blue[163] light. Your transforming crystal can be whatever size, shape, or color is right for you. Like healers, each one is uniquely beautiful.

In this variation, as you draw the pain into your hand, up your arm, and into your heart, it is transformed in the space between breathing in and breathing out. On the out-breath, the transformed pain flows back to the recipient as a soothing, beautiful blue light, all in one breath cycle. The nice thing about having it flow back to the recipient is that there is no emptiness or vacuum left where the pain used to be. You can fill that painful place with beautiful, soothing, comfortable blue light. This variation drains out the pain as you breathe in and fills the painful area with soothing, comforting light as you breathe out.

Drain the Pain Variation 2

This variation might be called *flushing* or *flooding the pain*. Rather than imagining draining (and replacing) the pain in step 3, in this variation, you simply flood the painful area with peaceful, comforting blue light[164]. With this variation, you anticipate that the pain will flow out of the recipient naturally all the way down to the feet and out into the earth, flooded and floated out by the healing, comforting light flooding in and replacing it. In this variation, the healer doesn't bring any of the pain into her body and doesn't try to transform it. She also doesn't use any of her own energy. She simply serves as a

---

163 For me and many other healers, blue is felt as a cooling, soothing, healing color. If you hate blue, and you find pink or lavender more soothing and comforting, use lavender. The point is to use your sensory imagination to create a strong sense of soothing, ease, and comfort, not to determine which particular shade of blue I'm thinking of. Similarly, I imagine the flow as light, but others may imagine it as water or silk or some other soothing substance.
164 Or the color and substance that feels most comforting to you.

channel to flood the painful area with so much universal positivity that everything else is washed away. I do not use this strategy very often because it can have a down side. If the pain is due to a blockage or a swelling (an accumulation or excess), adding more intensity could make things worse. Think of it this way: if you have a blocked drain in your sink, pouring a lot more water (even clean, clear water) in the sink could cause the sink to fill and water to cascade onto the floor as the sink overflows. You're better off draining the sink first and fixing the underlying problem rather than flooding it, hoping that the increased pressure will resolve things. If you see the problem as a fire that needs cool water to quench it, this approach might work, but if you see it as an accumulation or blockage, be careful about making things worse rather than better. In healing work, we rarely plan to achieve positive results by forcing or overwhelming something.

It's wise to make a plan with back-up options, continually re-assess, and change course when necessary. The third technique we'll practice is called Breaking Up the Blockage or the Ping-Pong Technique.

3. Breaking Up the Blockage (The Ping-Pong Technique)

I learned this technique from Rosalyn Bruyere, who is a very experienced healer. As the name implies, this is a vigorous strategy, and it should be used cautiously. I would not use this in a small child or a frail elderly person. I would not use it in someone with cancer, a serious infection, or rheumatoid arthritis. You might consider using it with an athlete whose pain is associated, not with acute inflammation or injury, but with chronic scarring that limits movement. Let's say for example, your thirty-year-old brother asks you for help with a frozen shoulder or your vigorous sixty-year-old aunt asks for help with a stiff elbow.

a. Begin as usual by taking a conscious breath, focusing on being centered and grounded; wash your hands; make sure the recipient is comfortable, and address things like the room temperature, sounds, light level, and privacy.

b. Assess the recipient. Ask where the pain or discomfort is worst, ask how severe it is on the zero-to-ten scale, and ask if it's okay to touch that area gently to ease the pain. Reassure the recipient that you can back off or touch the air over the area if it hurts too much to touch it directly, but that most people find this strangely soothing.

c. This is a two-handed technique in which both hands stay mostly still. Cradle the area that hurts between your hands, holding it gently. As with the foot-bone-to-anklebone technique, you will soon note a feeling of connection between your hands that most recipients feel as warmth.

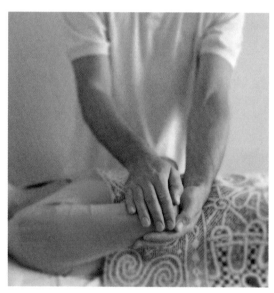

© **Nikki Zalewski – Fotolia.com**

Use your imagination to start sending soothing, healing energy from your dominant hand to your non-dominant hand, through the recipient's painful, stiff area. As soon as you feel it "ping" in the palm of your non-dominant hand, reverse the flow back to the dominant (now receptive) hand. As the receptive hand feels the soothing flow, it switches to sending. Imagine a Ping-Pong game happening between your hands with the recipient's body being the path along which the ball is pinging and ponging. You may start by having each "shot" from one hand to the other timed with breathing in, and the "shot" back timed with breathing out, but soon you will speed up so the Ping-Pong action occurs faster than your breath. Remain centered, grounded, curious, and neutral with regard to the outcome of this game.

Involve the recipient. Periodically ask the recipient how she notices the sensations changing. It might change from sharp to tingly or hot to full or magnetic or some other change. If at any point the recipient feels more uncomfortable, back off and switch to a more soothing technique (like #1 above).

I imagine a small, white Ping-Pong ball breaking up whatever is stuck, but your imagination may be different. You might imagine a plumber's plunger moving up and down, unclogging a drain, or a welder's torch melting a solid barrier. The goal is to remove a pain-causing blockage.

When you start to sense the blockage breaking open and moving, it's time to stop this particular technique and switch to soothing the area, pulling the blockage or congestion down and out. You are aiming for a balanced, harmonious sense of flow and ease throughout the body.

    a. Re-assess, remaining centered and grounded, with kind curiosity about the process and short-term outcome.

b. Finish, as usual, with your hands on the recipient's shoulders or feet, allowing her a rest period while you wash your hands and write some notes about the experience. Take a deep breath and return to your centered, grounded state.

The overall goal with healing treatments for pain is to promote a sense of flow, harmony, balance, order, and ease. You can help with your hands still or hands moving. Most often pain is associated with a sense of heat (inflammation) and the colors red and orange, so soothing images include light or water and the colors blue or green. The point is not to worry too much about the exact shade of color, but the feeling that color or image evokes in you. As a healer, your role is to use all your faculties, including your imagination, to generate a strong sense of well-being, peace, harmony, and comfort. It is as if you are using your inner Self as a tuning fork, generating a clear, pure note for the recipient to hum. You cannot sing for him, but you can make it easier for him to "sing" by resonating with his goal of increased comfort and ease, and the inner peace already present in his deepest self.

In the next chapter, we'll look at working with other common concerns—swelling, nausea, and constipation—before moving into working in pairs and working at a distance.

CHAPTER 15

Practices for Managing Edema (Swelling), Nausea, and Constipation

BY LEARNING HOW TO MANAGE STRESS, fatigue, and pain, you've learned to help the vast majority of people who are seeking healing. This chapter focuses on three important, but somewhat less common, situations: edema (swelling), nausea, and constipation.

What is Edema?

Edema is fluid accumulation in the tissues. The most common example is the swelling that occurs if you sprain an ankle. Edema occurs when more fluid leaks out of blood vessels (such as tiny capillaries and veins) than can be reabsorbed and returned via lymphatics to the heart. Sprained ankles typically have edema because the injury that causes the sprain also tears the tiny blood and lymphatic vessels in the ankle. Sprained ankles aren't the only cause of swollen ankles. Edema is also very common among women in the last months of pregnancy when the growing baby rests on and slightly blocks the blood flow in the veins returning blood to the heart, increasing pressure in the veins of the lower legs, leading to leaking fluid and

239

swollen feet and ankles. Edema can also be a sign of more serious conditions, such as kidney disease, heart failure, and hypothyroidism, liver disease, deep vein thrombosis, severe sepsis, or tumors. Edema is usually uncomfortable, and when it occurs over a joint like an ankle, it limits movement.

Regardless of the cause, healing treatment is geared toward restoring harmony, balance, flow, ease, and order to the system. Healers should remain centered and grounded, aware of their connection to their own inner stillness and harmony, while connecting to the inner self of the recipient and her capacity for balance and order. Healers should work with, not replace, conventional health care to ensure that any serious underlying illnesses are addressed. Remember, healers support and encourage the recipient's own healing process; healers do not claim to cure cancer, heart disease, or kidney failure.

a. Begin, as usual, by taking a conscious breath, focusing on being centered in your own sense of inner peace and grounded in your desire to relieve suffering and promote health and well-being; wash your hands; make sure the recipient is comfortable and that you've addressed things like the room temperature, sounds, light level, and privacy.

b. Assess the recipient. Observe how the recipient walks. If the swelling is in the feet, ask her to remove her shoes and socks so you can observe the skin (Is it tight and shiny, dull and pale, bruised, or something else?). Ask where the discomfort is worst, ask how severe it is on the 0 to 10 scale, and ask if it's okay to touch that area gently to ease the discomfort and swelling. Reassure the recipient that you can back off or provide a treatment without touching if preferred.

Make a plan. Most people start by working directly on the swollen area first (if that's what's bothering the recipient most), but some start with a whole-body treatment, soothing the stress (see Chapter 12) or increasing vitality (for those who are weak or debilitated; see chapter 13). Sometimes for frightened children, I start with the side that isn't hurting. For example, if a child has a right ankle sprain, I might start working on the left ankle so the child experiences my presence as safe and comforting and the process as comfortable and enjoyable. Starting with the healthy side also gives me an opportunity to become more familiar with what is normal or healthy for the child so I have a clearer sense of my goal with the hurting side.

One way to empower the recipient and help him feel more in control of the process is to offer choices. Offer simple choices in which you can easily live with either choice: do you want me to start with the right side or the left side? Do you want to keep your eyes open or closed? Do you want to be sitting up or reclining? Would you like me to prop your feet up? Are you warm enough? Would you like a blanket? Do you want the lights on or off? Would you like to listen to music, nature sounds, or keep it quiet? Most health care professionals dive right in to the usual routine of asking questions, doing a physical exam and issuing commands (put this under your tongue, sit here, look there, hold still, breathe now, hold your breath, point to where it hurts, etc.), and ordering tests, which lead to a diagnosis and treatment plan. But your job as a healer is not to diagnose and not to dispense a medication; your job is to offer comfort, peace, and a sense of security, evoking and supporting the healing process within the recipient. Simply confirming how much power the person has by making her choices explicit (and respecting and acting on her choices) supports her ability to heal.

Your plan should include the part that is swollen AND the whole person. The order in which you work can be individualized. Let's say that you plan to start with his sprained ankle.

a. When working on the feet and the recipient is sitting in a chair, the healer can squat, sit on a very low stool, or sit on the floor. I usually sit on the floor with the person's foot in my lap. I don't mind sitting cross-legged on the floor, but in general, for swelling, the recipient feels better if the foot is elevated, so it's more comfortable for her if we get her onto an exam table or bed. Or if there are two chairs in the room, prop the foot on the second chair (with a pillow if possible).

Once the recipient is as comfortable as you can make her, start by re-assessing the ankle. Get a good feel for it. Compare it again with the other ankle. Then start sweeping the hands gently about two to six inches off the body toward the toes[165]. Maintain a sense that you are *moving out* the edema fluid and supporting a healthy, organized pattern of connective tissue and strong blood vessels as you repeat this sweeping motion. Be sure to include the entire swollen area and include the knee, but mostly focus on the ankle and foot. When someone sprains an ankle, he may also tense up the other muscles in the legs, back, belly, and shoulders on both sides of the body trying to protect the ankle or prevent another fall. He may be unaware of how tense those muscles are until you start working on them and he feels them relax. This is normal. Smoothing motions at a steady, rhythmic, calm pace help promote a sense of calm and

---

165 I know that edema fluid drains physiologically toward the heart, but for healing purposes, we drain the extra fluid away from the ankle, out toward the toes, and metaphorically into the earth.

ease that allows many forgotten muscles to relax and the breathing to become slow and steady. You might time your hand motions with his breath to create an overall sense of harmony and order.

Consider using your imagination: you might imagine the recipient's sprained ankle looking more like the healthy one—inside and out, with healthy bones, tendons, blood vessels, and connective tissue. Or you might imagine the swelling like an over-filled balloon that is gradually deflating, becoming less tense and rigid. If you sense spikiness or heat over the sprain, you can imagine softening, soothing, and cooling the area. The precise kind of visual, auditory, or kinesthetic imagery you use is less important than the overall sense of restoring order, balance, flow, and harmony.

Be patient. It often takes several minutes for the recipient to relax and feel more comfortable and for you to get a sense that the healing process has accelerated.

Continue to involve the recipient. Ask him to tell you each time the pain number (0 to 10) drops a number. Positive expectations exert powerful healing effects.

When your intuition tells you the time is right, switch to providing a whole-body technique like relieving stress or building vitality. If you want, you can assess and address the left top front part of the head, the "pain thermometer," before returning to the ankle and any other areas that need extra attention.

b. Re-assess the whole person, including the ankle; you may not see an immediate change in swelling during the session, but in my experience, you will observe a change of some kind—discomfort, color, posture, how the ankle is held, how the person rests and breathes. Ask him to slowly and gently move the foot to see how it feels to him now, and again rate his comfort level on the 0 to 10 scale.

c. I generally close by gently holding the recipient's toes or shoulders, letting him know quietly that he can rest here awhile and when he's ready, gently stretch fingers and toes, hands and feet, come back to an awareness of the room, and open his eyes. Some people are curious and keep their eyes open during a healing session, but most relax, close their eyes, and enjoy the unusual and subtle changing sensations.

Wash your hands and jot down your own notes about the session while the recipient rests. Remember, you do your best, and the healing is in the hands of the recipient. Maintain your sense of inner peace (centering), goodwill (grounding), and non-attachment. Ask for feedback so you can learn and continue to improve. If the comfort level is better, remind the recipient how he was able to achieve his goal. The person who improves is the true healer.

Variation 1 for Edema

Swelling in the feet is not always due to a sprain, of course. If the recipient reports a problem with the heart, liver, kidneys, or adrenal glands, pay special attention to the upper right side of the belly and chest as well as the mid-back areas when you do your assessment. All of these organs affect fluid and salt balance in the body, and you may want to focus some of your healing attention on them as well as the swollen feet and ankles[166]. These areas may not seem as "hot" or

---

166 Pp 153-154 Krieger D. *The Personal Practice of Therapeutic Touch*. 1993 Bear and Company. Santa Fe, NM.

"spiky" as a recently injured ankle, so your imagined intention may not rely as much on sending "cooling blue" or "soothing silky water" to the area. Some healers prefer to use more "energizing" imagery for chronic organ problems, such as green to the liver and heart, and gold or yellow to the kidneys, adrenals, and solar plexus. Similarly, whereas most healing for recent pain or injury uses a downward, calming, soothing motion, recipients generally feel that when healers move their hands upward toward (rather than away from) the heart, the sense is more energizing[167]. Whether your intention is more sedating or more energizing, please allow the recipient to rest after a treatment with the swollen areas elevated to promote physiologic drainage and an opportunity for the new, more harmonious, balanced, healthy pattern to set.

If the recipient is pregnant, encourage her to rest on her left side to relieve the pressure on the blood vessels that run up the right side of the belly under the baby.

Variation 2 for Edema

If you are working in an intensive care setting, you may encounter a patient whose whole body is swollen due to systemic infection (sepsis). This kind of swelling is usually a sign of a very serious illness requiring the highest level of conventional care. Use a whole-body technique, and be brief and gentle. Avoid over-stimulating the recipient. The most important thing healers can do in this setting is to bring a sense of calm, peace, harmony, and the confidence that everything that can be done is being done. Encourage and support all those on the team contributing to this person's healing process, including fam-

---

167 Be cautious with this. While many people find upward sweeps toward the heart energizing, some find them irritating and uncomfortable, like a cat getting its fur ruffled.

ily and friends. Consider asking a family member to bring a photo of the person when he was healthy and fix it to the wall over the head of the bed so that every person who comes in the room visualizes him as healthy and vibrant.

Years ago, when working in Seattle's wonderful Children's Hospital, I was asked to see a little girl with osteomyelitis of the right foot. Osteomyelitis is a serious infection of the bone, treated with powerful antibiotics given by vein over several weeks. She had just started her treatment, and her foot and ankle were swollen and red. She had a fever and was sitting on the bed with her dad, looking scared, tired, and uncomfortable. After introducing myself, I offered to try something that a nurse and a wise old woman[168] had taught me. It didn't hurt, but if she didn't want me to do it, I wouldn't, and if at any point she wanted me to stop, I would. She looked at her dad briefly who smiled with a "what have we got to lose" expression, so she nodded and said, "Go ahead." Breaking healer's rules[169], I skipped the assessment, took a deep breath to center and ground myself, and started right in on the foot. My concentration was total, clearing the heat and spikiness I felt in the foot; comparing it with the healthy foot; back to the problem area; and ignoring the rest of her body. Bearing in mind the admonition to treat children

168 Dolores Krieger, RN, PhD, and Dora Kunz
169 I'm not encouraging bad habits here, but following in the footsteps of my iconoclastic teacher, one of the inventors of Therapeutic Touch (TT), Dora Kunz, who used to say with a twinkle in her eye that she didn't do TT correctly and she was a bad teacher (though a very practical girl) and then laugh heartily.

briefly, I stopped after less than ten minutes, telling her I'd done as much as I could and getting ready to leave. Her face was slightly brighter and had more color. "That was cool," she said. "Will you come back tomorrow?" "If you want me to, I will," I reassured her. The next day when I arrived, she was bouncing excitedly in bed, quite a contrast to the day before. "She's here! Tell her, Daddy, tell her!" Her father told me that when the doctors caring for her infection examined her foot, the redness and swelling were gone, her fever was down, and her blood tests had normalized. "Wow," I said, "those were some great antibiotics they used! I'm happy for you!" Neither she nor her father credited the antibiotics, though I reassured them that they were really important. She asked for one more healing treatment, and spent only one more day (rather than the usual several days to weeks in the hospital) before going home to finish her treatment with oral antibiotics.

A few years later, I had another experience with healing work for swelling and infection in one of America's great children's hospitals.

One day at Boston's Children's Hospital, I was asked to see an infant who had been born with a large opening in the belly button area (omphalocele), which exposed her abdominal contents to germs in the air. She had undergone emergency surgery with outstanding pediatric surgeons to close the opening. That was twenty days earlier, and she'd been on the most powerful combination of antibiotics that were available, but the surgical site was still swollen and infected, and she hadn't gained any weight, despite getting fluid and nutrients by vein. The redness around the line of stitches extended three to four inches in every direction, which pretty much covered her whole belly. Her mother hovered at her side, vigilant and protective. I came with another doctor who was learning about healing. We asked the baby's mother if we could offer a healing treatment that wouldn't hurt the baby, and we'd stop any time she wanted us to. She agreed, standing right next to us to supervise. We stood for a moment in silence, our hands facing each other to center and ground together (see Chapter 16) before we started to work on the baby. We stood silently on each side of the crib, and gently extended soothing and comforting images through our hands about six inches above her body to ease the heat that felt like it was pouring out of the baby's tiny tummy. In less than ten minutes, we stopped[170] and told the mother (who was now resting in the bedside chair) that we'd be back the next day. When we returned, she greeted us enthusiastically as "the miracle workers!" We wondered what had happened. "The redness is nearly gone, her fever is down, and her white count is down!" she said. The other doctor and I looked at each other in disbelief, "Well," I offered, "maybe she just needed twenty-one days

---

170 Remember to treat babies and very sick people gently and more briefly than healthier adults.

of antibiotics instead of twenty days." We returned daily to offer treatments[171], and the baby gradually healed from the infection, gained weight, and eventually went home with her family.

Now that we've reviewed several approaches to addressing edema and swelling, let's look at some strategies for another common symptom: nausea.

Nausea

Just about everyone has experienced the discomfort of nausea. It can accompany motion sickness (the bane of astronaut training), pregnancy, anesthetic drugs used in surgery, chemotherapy, migraine headaches, food poisoning, stress, and viral infections.

Strategies to Prevent Nausea

In addition to conventional medicines and complementary approaches like SeaBands® and ginger, simple healing strategies may help head off

---

171 The nurses said that in the first week after we started coming, the only time the mother left the baby's side was when the baby's father was there or we were there to offer a treatment. She felt safe enough with us that she could relax her constant vigil and leave the bedside briefly. This is one of the most powerful benefits of offering healing. It helps people feel safe, trusting, and able to relax. Decreasing stress is an important part of what healers do. So often in busy hospitals, the staff have to spend their days measuring vital signs, drawing blood, administering medicines, asking about symptoms, adjusting equipment, changing dressings, and documenting all of that, and they don't have time for the gentle touch and healing presence that mean so much to patients and families. This constant busyness deprives health professionals of the rewards of seeing their patients feel better and feel grateful, safe, trusting, and connected and contributes to the epidemic of burnout that plagues professional health care today.

nausea when it's anticipated (e.g., before surgery, chemotherapy, or a long car trip)[172].

1. Prepare as usual: hand washing, centering, grounding, addressing environmental factors (temperature, light, sound, pillows, blankets), assessment, and planning.
2. Offer a soothing whole-body treatment to help ease the stress of anticipation.

With hands still, extend a sense of stability, strength, and harmony to the areas in the middle of the chest and the solar plexus. Since nausea is often a hot, rushed feeling, you may want to imagine extending cool, blue, soothing light into these areas. Then extend a sense of balance and stability to the upper chest and left upper belly[173]. If the recipient is sitting and you have access to the back, extend that same sense of strength, stability, and balance from the solar plexus to the kidneys. With the hands still, place both hands over the upper right belly, just under the ribs, and extend a sense of stability and vitality[174]. Finally, place your dominant hand over the solar plexus and your other hand on the recipient's knees or feet and imagine a strong, clear connection downward.

Use a strong sweeping motion downward from the solar plexus over the lower belly and into the ground; repeat for the back.

Re-assess and finish this healing session by holding the recipient's feet and encouraging him to exhale strongly through his feet. As with all healing sessions, let the recipient rest while you wash your

---

172 Krieger D, *The Personal Practice of Therapeutic Touch*, (Santa Fe: Bear and Company, 1993), 158–160.
173 Those who like to use color may wish to use a yellow-gold as a symbol of strength and stability.
174 Those who like to use color may wish to use an emerald green as a symbol of strength and soothing vitality.

hands, jot notes about the session, and then ask for feedback so you can continue to learn and grow. Remind the recipient of common-sense strategies to help the intestines to function at their best: drink plenty of fluids to stay hydrated and avoid rich, fried, or fatty foods in the twelve hours before the anticipated event.

Healing Someone Who Has Nausea

1. After nausea has already hit, the recipient may simply want to rest quietly or sit near the toilet alone. If she asks for treatment, focus on the above strategies, strongly connecting the belly to the ground and avoiding any upward movements.

2. In addition, you can use SeaBands®, which are elastic bands with small plastic bumps placed on the acupressure points on the wrist (P6, located on the palm side of the wrist, about 2 finger breadths closer to the elbow than the wrist creases). This is a well-known and effective form of acupressure. Alternatively, you can use your fingertips as a focused non-touch stimulus, circling them clockwise over the P6 point about one to two inches above the skin. Personally, I prefer acupressure with the elastic bands that can be left in place safely for many hours, but it's nice to know about alternatives.

Healing Someone Who Has Constipation

Constipation is one of the most common symptoms seen in hospitalized patients, which are often remembered as the PANICS-F (Pain, Anxiety, Nausea, Insomnia, Constipation, Stress, and Fatigue). Common-sense approaches like adequate hydration, high-fiber foods

KATHI J. KEMPER, M.D., M.P.H.

(dried fruit like prunes, whole grains, beans, seeds, and vegetables), avoiding constipating food and medicines, and simple non-prescription medications can work wonders. Healing approaches can help, too.

> Robin was aptly named. She was an avid bird-watcher and nature photographer, who also happened to have cystic fibrosis. At age forty, she was on the list for a lung transplant, but while waiting, she was frequently hospitalized for pneumonia and debilitating constipation. Her pneumonia made her cough so hard that her ribs had cracked; the pain of the broken ribs was so intense that it was hard to take a deep breath, which was not helping her pneumonia. Ordinarily, patients with this much pain would be given a narcotic pain reliever. But because narcotic pain medicines cause constipation, she needed another approach to help manage her pain. That's when I was called. After working with her chest and rib pain, I turned to her belly. She had received every kind of treatment available to cystic fibrosis patients with advanced disease and constipation without relief, and she was eager to try a safe healing technique. I did my best, gently circling my hands in the air above her belly, clockwise circles, imagining the flow of large intestinal contents making their way along the natural route out. I heard some stomach gurgling, but no immediate effect (other than general relaxation, sleepiness, and pain relief). However, when I returned the next day, Robin related that within an hour, she'd had the outcome she'd been seeking for her constipation.

Several weeks later, when she was re-hospitalized, she asked for me soon after she got to her room. Again, results within the hour. "Whenever you treat me, results soon follow!" she joked with me. High praise indeed.

The main lesson I draw from this experience is that for constipation, the imagery of flow and movement is important. As with nausea, I also imagine things moving downward and outward. I do not want to flood a congested area with any sense that things might back up farther. The main image is for movement downward and outward for both nausea and constipation.

Moving from Higher to Lower to Help Soothe Nausea and Constipation

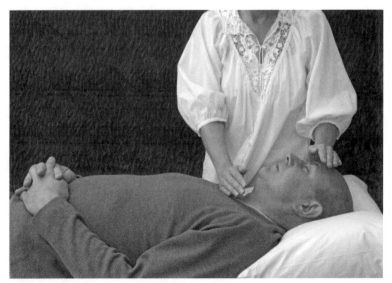

Move from higher - © Nikki Zalewski – Fotolia.com

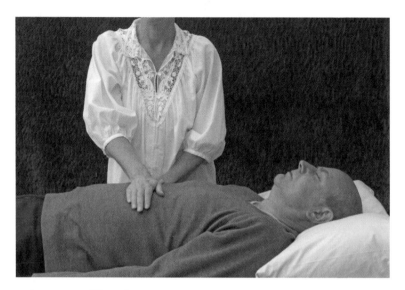

To lower - © Nikki Zalewski – Fotolia.com

We have covered the primary strategies for healing treatments addressing pain, anxiety, stress, or insomnia, nausea and constipation, and fatigue. The next chapter will help you do healing work with a partner.

CHAPTER 16

Strategies for Healing with Others—Working with a Partner

WORKING WITH A PARTNER OR GROUP of people to assist in the healing process offers both advantages and challenges. The advantages are significant: there is camaraderie, moral support, an opportunity for feedback and cooperative planning, and power in numbers. On the other hand, it requires skillful, flexible attention to focus on one's partner as well as the recipient; openness to hear feedback or perspectives that may differ from your own; humility to avoid trying to impress your partner; and self-awareness to keep the focus on the recipient and his needs rather than the relationship between healing partners. Once you and a partner or two outnumber the recipient, it's all too easy to turn him into a third party or a "case" rather than the central and most important person in the room. Remember, the true healer is the person who is going through the healing process—everyone else is a support person or facilitator.

In my experience, the advantages far outweigh the disadvantages in working with a partner or several partners. I usually work alone simply because of my clinical situation, but I enjoy and learn so much from working with others that I seek out partners whenever possible. That may be in part because that's how I was trained.

In both Therapeutic Touch and Healing Touch training, we usually worked in groups of two to three healers and one recipient at a time. Two of the healers would work directly with the recipient, sharing the tasks of centering, grounding, offering basic comfort measures (temperature, lighting, sound, aromas, posture, pillows) observation, planning, intervention, and post-intervention assessment, while the third or additional healers performed the task of "holding sacred space," being centered and grounded, and compassionately observing the entire interaction. Afterward, as the recipient rested, the observer could lead a brief, quiet discussion among the healers, hearing each one's observations and plans, interventions, and post-intervention assessments.

The observer has a unique perspective and can also provide feedback on how the interaction appeared to be between the healers—whether they were truly offering a harmonious, balanced, peaceful presence, or whether they seemed to be jockeying for power, waiting for someone to take charge, trying too hard, or distracted and mentally absent from the group. Just as the healers hold a compassionate attitude toward the recipient, the observer holds a compassionate attitude toward the recipient and the healers who are offering assistance.

May the Force Be with You

Remember Luke Skywalker? He learned to fly incredibly fast, complex maneuvers by allowing the Force to guide his intuition. In most of medicine, we give honor to rational, scientific materialism as the basis for our decision, yet most seasoned clinicians hold even deeper awe for the expert's "gut sense" or "clinical judgment." This is our way of saying that we value that hard-to-articulate inner knowing based on extensive, careful observation and deep experience. We value rational science *and* intuition.

> *"The intuitive mind is a sacred gift and the rational mind is a faithful servant."*
>
> —ALBERT EINSTEIN

Expanding Intuition to Include Partner as Well as Recipient

The main challenge in working with a partner is staying attuned to, and in harmony and balance with, the partner as well as the recipient, so it's helpful if you've had some experience with each other. Just as skilled musicians who know the same tunes can usually join a group and play together relatively easily, healers who are working from the same tradition and working for the same purpose (the recipient's well-being) can also generally work together effectively even if they've never met. The same is true for athletes playing team sports. For musicians and athletes, as well as healers, shared experiences and practice together over time lead to a beautiful, and at times uncanny, sense of harmony and intuition. If you are working with a close family member or friend, you may not need any exercises to develop a sense of attunement, but I have found it helpful to take a few minutes at the beginning of each session with a partner to attune with one another.

Let's try a few exercises to help you develop that sense of intuition together. The only thing you need is a willing partner and a sense of curiosity.

1. Push Me/Pull You

Remember Doctor Doolittle? This Disney movie included a two-headed llama called a pushmi-pullyu. In this exercise, you will work with a partner simply alternating the sense of pushing and pulling without touching your hands.

1. Begin by sitting or standing facing your partner with your eyes open. Take a deep breath and become centered in your inner sense of peacefulness and grounded in the desire for well-being for yourself and your partner.
2. Hold your hands up toward your partner a little below shoulder height and about three feet apart.
3. Slowly (over three to eight seconds) move your hands toward each other until they are only an inch apart. Now back off. Repeat two to three times so you get a sense of your partner through your hands as they approach each other. When do you start to feel her? Is it a sense of heat, cold, tingly, fullness, bounciness, magnetic feeling, buzzing, or what? There is no right or wrong answer. You are simply observing your partner's presence using your hands. Do you sense more strongly with one hand or another? Do you sense more easily with your fingertips or palms? Do you want to try with your eyes closed so you can concentrate more fully on the sensations in your hands? Go ahead.
4. Next, one partner holds her hands still while the other moves hands closer and farther away (pushing and pulling). The "hands still" partner can hold the hands upright as before (as if waiting for a high five) or hold them horizontally, palms open, as if getting ready to receive a box. The "push/pull" partner can imagine sending goodwill

as if it had a tangible quality like heat or cool, color or sound, texture or weight. Consider imagining goodwill as a sort of non-sticky ball of blue or pink cotton candy or a large, soft, white marshmallow or a big, green balloon or a warm loaf of bread or a cool autumn breeze. Pick ONE clear, vivid image to push into your partner's hands, and then gently pull it back, back and forth several times until you let it rest in your partner's open hands.

5. Briefly discuss what that was like for each of you. Then switch roles. Discuss again.

6. Now try the exercise one more time, but this time, do not move your hands. Decide which partner will start as the "push" partner and which will be the "pull" partner. The push partner will be palms down and the pull partner will keep palm(s) up, directly under the push partner's hands. Both partners keep hands still about three to six inches apart. Using your imagination, the "push" partner steadily extends a concrete image of goodwill into the "pull" partner's hands for about fifteen to thirty seconds. Stop. Discuss. Switch roles. Repeat. (Variation: try with just one hand.)

What did you notice? Was it easier to sense with hands moving or still? How far apart were your hands when you could easily sense your partner comfortably? Was it the same for both of you? Was it easier to sense pushing or pulling? How similar were the images each of you had while pushing/pulling? Don't worry about whether the images were similar. You

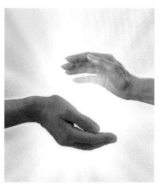

Push Pull Sensations © Nikki Zalewski – Fotolia.com

are just practicing using a type of sensation we usually ignore. Just as with listening through a stethoscope it takes a bit of practice to hear anything other than pounding of your own blood in your ears, it will take a bit of practice to feel anything through your hands.

For me, it took about three years to feel anything in my hands. And it took about another two years to feel confident that what I felt had any particular meaning. Others take to this right away with a high degree of intuitive accuracy. Remember, there are no studies showing that those who have more sensory awareness in their hands are more comforting and helpful than those who have different kinds of intuition. The main thing is to maintain a sense of inner peace and compassion toward the person you are trying to help. Don't get so focused on your own sensations or lack thereof that you forget why you're here.

2. Observer Intuition

When you are working with a partner, your observations include what you sense in your hands as well as what you see, hear, and feel in your body. When you serve as the observer, your hands are usually in your lap, so your observations and your intuition and assessment have one less type of input. Ready to test it?

1. Work in groups of three or more. Two people will serve in the "push" and "pull" roles, and everyone else will serve as observer.
2. Everyone starts by taking a few seconds to become centered and grounded. Everyone here is dedicated to becoming a more effective healer and helping others become more effective, too. Maintain the balance of peacefulness, kindness, and curiosity.

3. The person in the "push" role will lead. Again, the "pusher" has hands out, palms down and is hovering three to six inches above the "puller," who has hands out, palms up. The "pusher" decides on ONE image of loving-kindness, compassion, or goodwill to push to the recipient. It should include a color, texture, and/or temperature and be as vivid as possible. Extend that image for about thirty seconds. Relax.

4. This time, the observer starts the conversation. What did you observe? What's your best guess about the image being "pushed"? Observers guess before the "puller" (who had the advantage of sensing through the hands). Finally, the "pusher" describes the image of loving-kindness, compassion, or goodwill he was actually trying to "push." Enjoy the experience of guessing together.

5. Switch roles. The "pusher" becomes an observer; the "puller" becomes the "pusher," and the observer becomes the "puller." Repeat the entire experience including the discussion. And then switch roles again so everyone gets an opportunity to play each role.

What did you observe? Which role felt most comfortable for you? Which sensory modality was easiest for you to guess—visual, texture, temperature, or something else? What kind of feedback was most helpful to you? Don't worry if you couldn't feel or sense anything as the observer or puller. The most important thing is to remain centered in the peace and compassion in your heart and extend peace, kindness, and goodwill to others.

Before moving into actually working with a recipient, consider repeating some of the exercises from earlier chapters with a partner or two. For example, one person can offer the foot-bone-to-anklebone exercise to another while a third person observes. Or one can extend soothing sweeping motions from head to toe for another while an observer offers feedback on the speed and distance. These are opportunities for you to gain experience in knowing yourself and developing your intuition, not to judge yourself or others. Just as musicians and athletes set regular practice times with their performance partners, you may find it helpful to set regular practice times with your healing teammates.

Working in Pairs with a Recipient

When you're ready to work with a recipient, here are some easy steps to follow; start with common sense:

Both partners should introduce themselves to the recipient (and each other), be responsible for ensuring the recipient is comfortable, and wash their hands.

1. Both partners should take a few seconds to become centered and grounded before aligning with each other. This alignment is usually done by standing quietly with hands facing each other a few inches apart for a bit until both partners feel connected and in harmony with each other. Most pairs will soon find themselves breathing in the same slow, comfortable rhythm.

2. If the recipient is sitting, assessment is done with one partner in front and the other standing behind the recipient. Complete the observation and assessment from head to sitting bones (if in back) or head to toe (if in front). If the recipient is reclining, one partner generally observes and assesses from the right side while the other works from the left. Then switch positions so both partners can observe

and assess the whole person. Quietly make a plan together. Remember, healers do not diagnose. You should not say things like "well, this is really depleted," or that is "hot and inflamed," or "the liver needs attention," or "the hip feels cold," or anything else that might make the person feel worse or worried. Decide together quietly who will work on the front or back, the right or left sides. Feel free to ask the recipient how he is overall (use the 0 to 10 scale so you can compare before and after senses of pain, stress, fatigue, relaxation, well-being, or whatever seems appropriate) and ask if there's a particular part of the body that would like special attention. Agree to offer a focus on that area as well as overall well-being.

Make a plan together about what kind of approach you will use.

3. You can combine approaches, but be sure to coordinate. If one partner is making sweeping, soothing downward motions to offer a sense of calm and peacefulness, the other partner should mirror that. If one partner is using a foot-bone-to-anklebone process with hands still to build a sense of strength and vitality, the other partner can mirror this on the other side of the body. If one partner is draining the pain with hands still, the other partner can offer hands still on the mirror side of the body or simply hold the feet or shoulders to help promote an overall sense of well-being.

Both partners should maintain a sense of peace, kindness, and openness to the process and be aware of one another and your shared purpose. If your partner is still working when you feel finished, gently hold the recipient's feet or shoulders, continuing to extend peace and goodwill while your partner finishes. If you feel it is appropriate to do so, you can switch positions so you both have an opportunity to address right/left or front/back. If the recipient is a young infant, a restless toddler, or a very frail or debilitated person, you will likely want to keep the treatment brief, so you will probably not switch sides.

1. When you both feel finished, take a moment to repeat your assessment. Ask the recipient again if there's any other part of his body that needs a bit more attention and ask him to again rate his primary concern on the 0 to 10 scale.

2. Let the recipient know you are finished and he can take a few minutes to rest while you both wash your hands and make some notes for yourself and in the recipient's health record if appropriate (only one of you needs to write in the health record). Again, check to make sure the recipient is comfortable. Offer to get him some water if he's still awake. Offer thanks to each other and to the recipient for the opportunity to do this work together.

If the recipient falls asleep in a hospital, hospice, or home setting, thank your partner. Leave a note for the recipient, thanking him for the opportunity to work together and letting him know if and when you will return. If the recipient has another caretaker (a nurse, family member, or friend) who is caring for him, check in with that person to let them know you were there, what you did (avoiding technical jargon), and how the recipient responded. Be a good team member—communicate with others on the team. Offer encouragement and support, and do not claim personal credit for any outcome.

If you are in a hospital room or exam room, step outside and close the door to discuss the session quietly. If you are in an open area, avoid whispering your observations or comments to each other in earshot of the recipient. It is simply human nature for the recipient to wonder what you are saying about him and to wonder if it's something bad. Do not add to the recipient's worries or stress.

If the recipient is awake, offer some anticipatory guidance. This means to let the recipient know what to expect over the next few hours. It is normal for people to feel pleasantly drowsy after a healing session. Some people who have been fatigued feel energized for several hours afterward. Sometimes people don't notice much at the time, but they find their sleep more restful or deep the night of a healing session. Whatever the recipient experiences is normal for them. Offer to answer questions, but remember to avoid making a diagnosis. Keep your answers simple and hopeful.

Ask whether he would like to plan another session and when it would be convenient, or if he'd like to think about it and get back to you. Do not pressure the recipient to plan more sessions. But do be available and reliable. If either of you is about to go on a trip and will not be available, offer the name of another person you trust as a healer, or inform the recipient when you will return, or offer to do a solo session if desired. When someone has offered to be vulnerable to you and has allowed you the intimate opportunity to serve in a healing capacity, you want to honor that trust. Return to your sense of inner peace and compassion.

That's a simple summary of what do to when working with a single partner. But what do you do when there's more help available?

Working with More than One Partner

Whenever there's another person present for the healing process, that person is involved in the process, too. So, if you and a partner find yourself in a room with a recipient and one or more other people, get them involved.

Sometimes I will ask bystanders to take concrete action consistent with their beliefs. I ask them to call a prayer line or pray; hang a "do not disturb" sign on the door; adjust the blinds or lights; pour a glass of water; pull a privacy curtain; or turn off the television. Even small children can be asked to draw a pretty picture to cheer the recipient. Everyone likes to feel useful, and being able to do something usually makes people feel better, stronger, and more hopeful, which creates a helpful atmosphere for healing.

If the other person wants to be involved and do something else, I usually ask them to watch for a few minutes so they get a sense of what's going on, and then hold the recipient's feet to help them feel safe, secure, and grounded. If they feel comfortable using their imagination, I might ask them to imagine breathing in the strength of Mother Earth through their feet, as if they were oak trees with deep roots, drawing strength, stability, and nutrients from the earth, and breathing that strength out through their hands into the recipient's feet. If you have two people who want to be involved, assign a foot to each one.

The easiest way to be involved requires no special training or imagination. It simply means staying present, finding the most peaceful part of one's inner self, and extending goodwill, kindness, and the wish for well-being to all those involved in caring for the recipient. As a professional caregiver, I'd much rather be in a room with someone extending goodwill and kindness than someone who is simply reading the newspaper with its daily dose of "if it bleeds, it leads." If you're lucky enough have a crowd of volunteers, ask them to create a circle around you, your partner, and the recipient, and extend goodwill to everyone inside the circle.

Communication

When working in pairs or groups, communication is paramount. You may like the room dim, whereas your partner may want it bright. You may like music, whereas your partner prefers silence. You may not like scents, whereas your partner adores aromatherapy. Be open with each other, listen respectfully, and always defer to the recipient. If the recipient doesn't care about some aspect of the environment, but it matters to you, let your partner know. There are very few deal-breakers when it comes to differences in healing styles, environments, or techniques, but festering resentment is a surefire way to hurt a partnership. It's far better to get disagreements or preferences out in the open than foster misunderstanding or martyrdom.

Language

> *"The United States and Great Britain are two countries separated by a common language."*
>
> —George Bernard Shaw

Don't let language differences come between you and your partner. I have worked with other healers trained in shamanism, Therapeutic Touch, Healing Touch, acupuncture, Polarity Therapy, and Reiki, as well as spiritual healers from a variety of faith and spiritual backgrounds. Each healing tradition uses its own language, imagery, and metaphors to describe the process used for healing. Some call it love; some call it beauty; some call it energy, chi, or prana. As my friend and colleague, Deborah Larrimore, likes to say, "Regardless of what you call it, it's all the same energy."

As a medical professional, I try to avoid the word "energy" because it conjures up physics classes and physical energy for most biomedically trained professionals. Since I don't know exactly what kind of physical energy or information is being transferred during healing work, I prefer to use words like compassion, healing presence, comforting presence, peace, goodwill, and loving-kindness. As a scientist, I'm also comfortable admitting there are many things that have not undergone sufficient research. Even though love, healing, and beauty remain mysteries, they are also powerful forces in our human experience. Let's use our common humanity and shared goals for healing to bridge the differences that at times seem to divide us.

PART 4

Final Thoughts

CHAPTER 17
Distant Healing

As a biomedical researcher, I have really wrestled with whether or not to include this chapter. The scientific evidence for the effectiveness of distant healing is mixed. Distant (or non-local) healing has powerful advocates and powerful critics, both of who fiercely defend their positions with loads of logic and data. Why would I want to put myself in the middle of this controversy?

Integrity. I reflected on the reasons I started to write this book, and I realized that this chapter had to be included. The reason I started this book was to write the book I wish had been available when I started medical school. And to be honest, to come completely out of the closet about my interest in healing, I have to admit that despite the mixed and contradictory evidence, despite the mystery surrounding any possible mechanism for its effectiveness, I engage in distant healing work.

In fact, much of my interest in healing started before I decided to go to medical school. It happened one day when I was a teenager, surrounded by friends, during a particularly deep group meditation. Here's what happened.

One day in the summer of 1974, I was visiting my godmother in Virginia Beach. She taught about meditation and Jungian-style dream interpretation, and usually had several friends visiting. We had many lively, laughter-filled, and serious discussions around her kitchen table. One day we were talking about a friend's health problem and how if we were alive during New Testament times, Jesus might heal her. As twilight fell, I had a strange experience. As I listened to everyone talking, I felt as if I were floating out of my body and had a high-speed review of my entire life with a loving guide who showed me the patterns and lessons in my experiences. I went to the living room to meditate and absorb this information while the moon rose over the water. The loving guide who had shown me my life patterns re-appeared with several similar beings in the background and silently asked what else I would like to know. I asked how Jesus healed. Rather than tell me an answer in words, the guides simply showed me a series of images. One of them showed me "her" body with a physical problem. "Now watch," they seemed to say. The solid physical body appeared to shift to a less substantial, more subtle body, but the problem was still visible. It appeared to shift again, to something even less substantial. Each time the body had its same general form, but it became more amorphous, less solid, and as it did so, the problem seemed to grow less substantial, too. Finally, there was only a barely visible pattern of waves, as if you might be able to see radio waves in the general form of a human body. At this point, there was no physical problem. The problem had first appeared at one step below this level, at a vibration or level of slightly greater solidity. I was given to understand that there were two easy ways to heal. Both involved a shift in ordinary awareness. First, go to the awareness of the very highest level of being where there is no problem and affirm with the person that "perfection" so that it resonates down through every level of being until it manifests in the most solid, physical form. Second, go to the awareness of the level where the problem first appears and it is easily corrected or removed and do that, knowing that the correction will be amplified on each subsequent level until it reaches the solid physical form where it will no longer exist. Whatever is corrected on the higher levels of awareness will be manifest at the lower levels. As above, so below. It sounds simple, but I wanted to know more. I'd never heard of anything like this. "Who will teach me to do this back in my normal state of consciousness?" I wondered. The guides seemed to smile with gentle reassurance that I needn't worry about that.

This experience was even more mysterious to me because I was a healthy teenager, and like most healthy teenagers, I took good health and vitality for granted and was not particularly interested in health or healing. I was planning to study physics and had grand plans to work on the problem of cold fusion so we could avoid future energy crises. I had no idea that after I went to college, my career plans would change several times before I ended up in medicine.

After I'd made the decision to study medicine, I met Dr. Gladys McGarey, one of the founders of the American Holistic Medical Association, the mother of integrative medicine. I asked her which medical school would teach me about the kind of healing I'd seen in that vision in 1974. She laughed and said there were no medical schools teaching healing, but I should go to medical school anyway because it would be useful for other things. "How odd!" I thought. "What other things could be more important?" But indeed, I have learned many useful things; seen the astonishing power of modern medicine to cure and manage serious disease; and witnessed the incredible dedication, kindness, and self-sacrifice of so many doctors, nurses, therapists, and staff who work in modern health care settings.

After completing medical school, a master's degree in public health, three years of residency training in pediatrics, and two years of research fellowship training, in 1989 I attended my first Therapeutic Touch workshop with Dora Kunz. At that workshop, I felt that I was finally learning about the second type of healing I'd envisioned in 1974.

But I had actually witnessed an example of the first type of healing back in college.

During a friendly game of football, one of our classmates took an unexpectedly hard hit and clearly had a broken arm, which was hanging at an odd angle. He was very groggy, but we managed to get him to the emergency room, where X-rays confirmed the fracture. As we waited with him for the orthopedist to set his arm, our friend finally woke up fully and came to himself. "Where am I? What am I doing here?" he asked frantically. We tried to explain, but he insisted on leaving. "I'm a Christian Scientist," he insisted. "I don't believe in all this. I have to go pray. And I have to call my parents and my church so they can pray, too." We thought

> he was nuts, but the next day, his arm was absolutely fine. None of us had any reasonable scientific explanation other than doubting our own experience the day before.

Obviously that experience did not dissuade me from pursuing a career in modern medicine. I did not become a Christian Scientist, and I do not avoid medications, vaccinations, or surgery.

Remember the four dragons from Chapter 6? It is dangerous to delude ourselves and deny what is happening, hoping that by simply affirming what we wish were true, we will make it true.

"We cannot solve our problems with the same level of thinking that created them."

—Albert Einstein

We cannot simply wish our symptoms away. We cannot simply fantasize our problems into oblivion. Reciting platitudes does not reverse pathology. Modern psychology has taught us the enormous power of our unconscious mind. Even if we tell our conscious mind that "everything is okay," if our unconscious mind thinks otherwise, the unconscious prevails.

My vision of healing (whatever its source) indicated that healing happens only when our consciousness, our awareness, shifts into a different, higher state. We cannot remain in the same level of thinking and solve the problem.

So, when I engage in distant healing, I start by meditating to shift my consciousness to another level of awareness, a level where we are all connected to one another. This is not ordinary consciousness. It is not a mealtime wish list: "Thank you for this food. Please bless

Grandma and Grandpa, and help Mr. Wilson's sciatica. Amen. Pass the potatoes." I am all for prayers of gratitude and thanksgiving, but squeezing in a healing wish between bites as if making a magical Christmas list is not a powerful approach to healing.

Here are the steps I use when I engage in distant healing:

1. Become centered in the stillness within and the sense of connection to the Creative Forces and the one seeking healing. Become grounded in loving-kindness and compassion, the deep desire that all experience well-being and relief of suffering.

2. From this sense of connection, assess the recipient. Please remember that whether you are working in person or at a distance, it is generally considered unethical to intervene without permission. Yes, of course, you can pray for peace in the Middle East and the end of starvation for all children everywhere without a specific request from an individual, but when you decide to focus on an individual, other than a public official, outside of an emergency, ask before assessing or intervening. How do you assess at a distance? It requires focused attention and imagination, a shift from ordinary awareness. I imagine the person sitting, standing, or reclining in front of me, and I observe as if we were physically together. Some healers can do this with just a name and location, but it's much better for me if I've met and worked with a person in person before attempting healing work at a distance.

3. At this stage, you have a choice. If you are able to shift your awareness to higher and higher levels until you reach the point that the recipient is completely whole and well,

do that. Hold that image, and then carry it downward through each level, pausing and going back up a level if you start to "see" a problem, and again holding that image of wellness down through each level until you reach "normal" awareness. If you are unable to shift your awareness to higher levels, that's okay, just work with the person as if she were with you. Remember the general rules: "If there's stress, calm it. If there's pain, soothe it. If there' fatigue, revitalize it. If there's imbalance, balance it. If there's chaotic scattering, restore a sense of order. If there's fullness, drain it. If there's emptiness, fill it." Work until you feel a sense of completion. It may be one minute. It may be twenty minutes. Trust your intuition.

4. Re-assess the whole person.

5. Release the person to complete his or her own healing process. Come back to your ordinary state of awareness. I usually give thanks for the opportunity to be present with another person on her healing journey. I also usually wash my hands, which may simply be a symbolic gesture for me to release the experience before moving on to the next activity. Return to your sense of peace and compassion.

6. "Trust, but verify." I also usually see or call the recipient later on to find out how she is doing. It's good to have regular reality checks to avoid getting lost in fantasy land.

Does Distant Healing Work?

As I mentioned at the beginning of this chapter, the scientific jury is still out on this. But I will tell you a story that helped convince me that doing this work is worthwhile.

At Boston Children's Hospital, I was asked to see a teenager who had developed a rare, but serious, infection in his blood stream and liver. Jacob was desperately ill in a coma in the intensive care unit (ICU). His family wanted a healer. The staff called me. I worked with him daily for several days, not seeing any response—no change in heart rate, breathing, oxygen levels, nothing. He remained comatose. I was scheduled to leave town on business for several days and told Jacob's family I'd look for him when I returned. While I was gone, I decided to continue our sessions each night after my family had gone to bed. So, at ten p.m., I'd sit quietly, do distant healing work with Jacob, wash my hands, and go to bed. When I returned to Boston, I went to see him. Jacob had markedly improved and moved out of the ICU and into a regular hospital bed on a different ward. I knocked on the door and prepared to introduce myself. This was the first time I'd seen Jacob awake, and I was eager to see him now that he could talk. But he interrupted before I could speak. "I know who you are," he beamed. "You're the doctor who comes to see me every night at ten p.m." His mom looked confused. "I thought you were out of town," she said. "I was," I replied, "but he was so sick that every night I continued to do healing work with him after the rest of the day's work was finished."

"I knew you were here," Jacob said, "you started coming in the ICU, and you kept coming even after I moved and all the other doctors and nurses changed. You look just like yourself, even in person."

I was astonished. How had he recognized me? His eyes had been closed; he'd been in a coma. He hadn't heard me because I hadn't spoken out loud in his presence in the ICU. There were no pictures of me in his room or posted anywhere in the hospital. Yet, somehow, the connection forged on those other levels of awareness had percolated through his consciousness, and he knew me down to my physical appearance.

Since then I've had many other experiences working with friends, family, and patients at a distance. Often recipients have reported that they felt better at the moment I was miles away concentrating on our healing work together. Yet none have been as dramatic as Jacob.

Do we need more research? Of course, I'd like to have a lot more scientific data on how to heal at a distance effectively and consistently. In the meantime, I'll trust my experience and try to learn from each encounter. What will you do?

The next chapter gives you additional tips on how to empower a recipient's continued healing between sessions.

.

CHAPTER 18

Homework—Wellness
Practices between
Healing Sessions

ALTHOUGH HEALING FOR ACUTE CONDITIONS can sometimes occur quickly, recovery from chronic, long-standing conditions usually takes longer. If a condition is the result of a habit, such as smoking, sedentary living, poor diet, intemperate use of alcohol, or emotional patterns of fear, anger, envy, or blame, additional actions are needed, not just to recover, but to reduce the risk for future disease. Even short-term conditions may benefit from interventions in addition to your healing work. Here's an example from a patient I saw recently.

Frances was a sixteen-year-old girl referred to me for treatment of chronic abdominal pain and headaches. After doing my usual review of her medical chart and talking with her and her family about conventional and complementary therapies, I asked if she'd like to try something right in the moment to help ease her pain. Since her pain was an eight out of ten, she readily agreed to try. Within a few minutes,

281

her belly pain and headache were completely gone. But she still reported a pain level of 5.5. Why? The tip of her left index finger was red and swollen, and it appeared to be infected around the base of the nail where she'd been chewing on a hangnail (Always do a complete assessment, I reminded myself!). So, we took a few minutes to address the finger pain. Again, the pain receded within a few minutes, and remarkably, the swelling and redness had noticeably diminished, too. We were all delighted! But this didn't mean we were through. I advised her to soak the finger in hot water, apply an over-the-counter antibiotic ointment, and do the things we'd discussed in terms of her sleep, diet, medications, and other therapies. Homework!

Homework can help establish new, healthier patterns of living. It can be a short-term activity like soaking an infected finger or changing a long-term habit like eating fewer chips and more vegetables. It doesn't need to be dramatic. Sometimes making a series of small shifts over time can lead to more sustainable changes toward a healthy lifestyle than major changes. Going to bed fifteen minutes earlier at least four days a week is a lot easier to do than going to bed two hours earlier and expecting to do it daily. Setting achievable goals sets a pattern for success that makes other changes easier. Remember, Rome wasn't built in a day.

One of the trickiest parts of suggesting homework is to empower someone to make healthy choices while avoiding the "blame the victim" game. Guilt is debilitating. Avoid inducing it. One of my mentors, Dr. Abe Bergman, used to tell me that the pediatrician's most important job was "to be a cheerleader for mothers." That's great advice! And not just for mothers. Of course, mothers tend to feel guilty when their children are sick or injured, and mothers worry that health professionals, other mothers, and THEIR mothers will think they are not doing a good job. All that worry can be self-defeating. Worry is not healing. Rather than tell moms (or others) not to worry, it's far more helpful to notice all the things they are doing well, praise their loving intentions, and encourage them to trust their intuition and their good judgment.

Another one of my mentors, Dora Kunz, frequently gave practical homework after a healing session. Her homework suggestions fell into three main categories:

1. Self-talk
2. Self-care
3. Other-care

Let's review a few examples of each kind of homework Dora recommended.

Self-Talk Homework

It's very common for people suffering from a chronic illness or the long-term effects of an injury to start to identify themselves with their problem. They develop a mental picture of themselves:

"I am a cancer patient."
"I am a pain patient."
"I am an accident/trauma/violence victim."

This kind of mental picture limits our identity to the problem. While it may be true that a person is in the role of a patient, most people have multiple roles, and limiting identity to just one of them makes the problem dominate their consciousness. Instead it's helpful to think:

"I *have* ____(a disease)____. But I am more than my disease."
"I *have survived* ____(trauma)____. And I am more than that experience."

Switching from "I am" to "I have" is a small shift, but it can have powerful effects on our self-perception. We are more than our symptoms—a lot more.

If the symptom isn't constant, it is helpful to emphasize its temporary nature.

"I *sometimes* have pain. But I am more than the pain."

Or if the symptom is present in the moment:

"I *have* pain *in this moment*. But I am more than the pain."

Including the time element in the statement implies the possibility that the symptom or condition will change, and that implies the possibility of improvement.

Frances had told me that her belly pain was constant, that nothing made it better or worse, and that it was even present when she was asleep. Her clinic questionnaire showed that her family had just welcomed a new little nephew for her. "What happens to your pain when you see and hold baby Joey?" I asked her. "Oh, I feel a lot better. Here, you want to see some pictures?" She pulled out her mom's phone and started showing me pictures of adorable Joey. Her face lit up like Christmas. "Wow," she noted, "just looking at his pictures makes me feel better." She also realized that the pain was worse when she drank milk. Within a very short time, she was able to identify several things she could control that made her pain either better or worse. And she was on the road to feeling more powerful than the pain.

The point of this kind of conversation is to help empower a person like Frances so she has more energy to overcome adversity and to make changes to improve her well-being. Back to self-talk homework . . .

It can also help to make a third tiny shift as we talk to ourselves. Shift from "I" to using your name, as if you are talking about yourself.

"Frances has ____(pain)____. But Frances is much more than the pain. Frances is a student, an aunt, a cat owner, a photographer, and much more."

"John Doe has survived ____(trauma)____. And John is more than that experience."

Talking about yourself in the third person creates a sense of objectivity. Particularly for people who habitually judge themselves harshly, talking about themselves in the third person can make it easier to be friendly and kind to themselves. Listing a variety of roles helps lift us out of the victim role and reminds of things that are important to us. This kind of self-talk is uplifting and energizing.

The goal of this self-talk homework is to help shift self-perception from the limited illness or injury to a more neutral or even positive perspective. Here is a true statement that does not deny the reality of the person's experience of having a disease or condition:

"Frances is more than her pain, and she has the potential for order, wholeness, harmony, peace, kindness, and well-being."

Try this homework yourself at least five days in the next week. Stand in front of a mirror, and using your own name, say:

"MY NAME is more than her condition, and she has great potential for order, wholeness, harmony, peace, kindness, and well-being."

Before you recommend homework to someone else, it's helpful to have done it yourself. This will help you anticipate the barriers and resistance that someone else might have in starting a new self-talk program. Go ahead. Sit or stand in front of a mirror and talk about yourself positively. How does it feel? How does the experience change with repetition?

Self-Care Homework

In our busy world, many people are too busy with work, school, household chores, and family and community responsibilities to take the time to care for themselves. Being sick or in pain is a good reminder that in all our "busyness," we can be more effective in the long run if we care for ourselves. Here are a few suggestions.

1. Take some time to go outside and appreciate nature. Visit a tree, a garden, or a park, green space, stream, or other body of water. Evergreen trees can be particularly soothing since they maintain their greenery even in the depths of winter. Spending time in nature is restorative.
2. Throughout the day, at least once or twice, take a few deep, cleansing breaths. Taking a few deep, slow breaths is like

hitting the reset button of our autonomic nervous system. Doing it when you're NOT stressed helps your body stay calm and collected so when something stressful happens, you respond from a more peaceful perspective.

3. Eat something wholesome and nourishing. Sometimes we lose our appetite when we're ill, but even then, we can plan to have a few sips of healthy broth. Taking a few sips or bites of small meals throughout the day may be easier when we're ill than trying to force down three large meals, and it helps us keep a more even blood sugar and remain hydrated, both of which help us feel better.

4. Take a nap. You may not have napped since you were a toddler, but when you are sick, taking a twenty-minute catnap may help restore your energy so you can get through the rest of the morning or afternoon. If you find that daytime napping interferes with your ability to fall asleep at night, then spend twenty minutes listening to soothing music.

Helping Others Homework

When we're sick or suffering, it's natural to turn inward and become self-absorbed. Some of us just want to be alone, curl up, and sleep. While that can be helpful for a short-term illness like the flu or a stomach bug, getting into that as a habit over weeks and months can lead to depression.

Several years ago, I saw Brian, a tall teenage boy with chronic fatigue who also seemed to be depressed. After having mono (when he was seriously fatigued and couldn't attend school), he'd gotten into the habit of sleeping late, skipping school, and heading to the basement to play video games for hours. He didn't socialize with any friends in person, he barely ate, and he didn't have many plans for the future. Exercise was one of the strategies we discussed to help restore his energy and attitude, but he claimed to be too tired, and anyway, he had not been much of an athlete before he'd gotten sick, so there was nothing much he wanted to do. So, after doing a healing session with him (and talking with his parents about other therapies), I gave him homework. "I want you to go down to the YMCA tomorrow and volunteer to help coach a basketball team," I told him. "But I don't play basketball, and I wouldn't be any good at it," he resisted. "Doesn't matter," I said. "Those kids need a bigger kid to look up to. That's more important than whether you know anything about basketball." His parents understood what I was trying to do for him and offered to drive him. When I saw him a month later, he was standing straighter, going to the Y three times a week to help, and attending school again. Was it the homework? We'll never know, but I do know that having a team of young kids look up to you and look forward to seeing you gives a person a reason to get out of bed. Actually getting out of the house regularly is also a reminder that there's more to life than the bed and the basement.

Doing things for others helps us feel better about ourselves, and like the self-talk exercises above, it helps us identify with a role other than the sick role.

The activity needn't be as demanding as volunteering three times a week. It can be something small like sending a card or a thank you note to someone else who needs cheering or who has offered a kindness. Simply reaching out to another can lift our spirits and build healing social relationships. Or it can be caring for a plant or pet.

A few years ago, I began caring for Rachel, a sixteen-year-old girl who suffered from chronic fatigue and moodiness; she had also lost her creative spark and had stopped attending school. She was not suicidal and would not see a psychotherapist for cognitive behavioral therapy, nor change her diet or start an exercise program. She did not want medications and took supplements sporadically. I suggested she might consider getting a dog that she could take for regular walks which would help her get outside in the sunshine, give her another source of unconditional love (both parents were loving and supportive), and provide her with an opportunity for regular exercise. Allergies in another family member ruled out this possibility. I was running out of ideas. Months later she returned to clinic with a bounce in her step and a gleam in her eye. What happened? Ducks! What? Her parents had gotten her baby ducks for Easter; she'd cared for them and they'd imprinted on her. She walked them to the creek behind their house daily in the morning and back to the garage in the evening. Caring for these baby ducks gave Rachel a new sense of purpose, confidence, and responsibility. They reminded her that she could make a difference, and that made a difference in her life. This was the first time I'd ever heard of duck therapy. But it worked. Homework can come in all shapes and sizes.

If you are a health professional, you may think of many more kinds of homework to aid the healing process. Whether you are a professional or a friend or family caregiver, consider these three simple types of homework exercise to extend the healing process:

- Self-talk
- Self-care
- Care for others

Any questions? That's what the next chapter is all about.

CHAPTER 19

Frequently Asked Questions (FAQs)

Q. *I'm a scientist, and I haven't seen this energy that so many healers talk about. It's hard to believe in healing when I don't believe in energy. Can I be a healer if I don't believe in "energy"?*

A. Yes. Although many healers describe their experience as one of assessing, channeling, or modulating energy, it is not necessary to believe in "energy" as anything other than a metaphor. It is far more important for you to become adept at centering yourself and maintaining that awareness of peace and harmony while extending it to another person with kindness and compassion than it is to adopt a particular belief system or language for describing your experience.

Q. *What about auras and the etheric, astral, and mental bodies?*

A. Many mystical traditions describe multiple levels or aspects of human existence. The lowest (or most dense) body is the physical body, which we can see, hear, smell, touch, and measure. The next level, closely associated with the physical body, is the etheric or vital body or body double. The next finer, less dense body, which is associated with emotions and emotional patterns, is called the astral body. Even more subtle is the mental body, the home of archetypal images and thoughts, intuition, creativity, and the level at which we can observe and interact non-locally. Some traditions describe even more subtle levels or layers. Each of the non-physical bodies has a field or energy that is described by very sensitive (clairvoyant) people as an aura. The different bodies are connected by energy centers, known as chakras. It is believed that illness or disease can originate at any of these levels and in fact may exist for some time on a subtle level long before becoming manifest physically. Instrumentation, such as Kirlian photography, is thought to be able to capture images of the vital/etheric body, but the ability to measure these bodies reliably and reproducibly with standard scientific instruments is controversial. Despite the abundance of historical experience suggesting these different aspects or levels of human existence, most modern scientists consider them metaphorical at best. As technology advances, we may find ways to measure the human energy field, or it may remain a helpful metaphor. Being aware of your own inner sense of peacefulness and the capacity for peace, harmony, and well-being in others is more important than being able to see or measure auras.

Q. I've tried to feel that energy that people talk about, but I don't feel anything. My hands get tingly, but I think that's just my circulation or my nerves. Sometimes I feel warmth, but that's probably just blood flow. Can the healing I offer do any good if I don't feel energy?

A. Yes. In fact, if you try too hard to feel something, you are likely to distract yourself from remaining centered and grounded. Distractions limit your effectiveness. So, don't worry so much about what you feel in your hands as what you feel in your heart. Practice the paradox of remaining centered yourself while extending your awareness to another person and connecting to their center of stillness, wholeness, and harmony. Your outer sensory perceptions are less important than your inner motivation and centering. On the other hand, pay attention to what your recipient tells you. And if you're a health professional, do not disregard the symptoms, signs, laboratory tests, and imaging studies that inform your thoughts and actions.

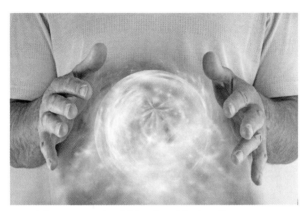

Imagining Energy © Nikki Zalewski – Fotolia.com

Q. I'm working with someone who seems to relax, but I'm not sensing an impact with my hands. Should I just try harder?

A. No. If you are working with someone, but are not sensing an effect, it is better to stop than to try harder and possibly overwhelm or irritate the recipient. Re-center yourself. Ask for feedback from the recipient or ask another healer or health professional for help. Healing is an effortless effort.

Q. I just don't feel that confident. What should I do?

A. Practice with others who are learning and those who are generally healthy and robust. Gain experience with simple practices, such as:

- Hands still, allowing goodwill to flow from your hands into a recipient's back over the kidneys/adrenal

- Hands still, holding the recipient's feet while you imagine energy flowing from the earth up into your feet, your heart, your hands, and energizing the recipient
- Hands moving about two to three inches above the body, moving steadily and rhythmically down from the head/center to the feet/periphery.

Do not practice with vulnerable patients when you feel uncertain or lack confidence. Recipients will sense your lack of confidence just as a horse senses an inexperienced rider. Patients who are vulnerable, very sick, very young, or elderly can pick up your non-verbal cues and feel worse, more anxious, or that they need to make an effort to reassure you rather than simply relax in a trusting relationship. Practice with healthy family members and colleagues to gain confidence. Give yourself time. You can do it.

Q. What if I get distracted during a treatment?

A. Good for you for being self-aware enough to notice when your mind wanders. If you get distracted during a treatment, take a breath, return to being centered and grounded, and start over. Do not mechanically wave your hands around. Consider practicing meditation regularly to help build your concentration.

Q. I've seen healers shake their hands while treating someone, as if they are trying to shake off bad vibes. Can healers catch diseases from those they are treating?

A. Good observation. Healers can catch viruses and bacteria just as anyone can from another person. Good hygiene (covering sneezes, washing hands with soap and water, washing sheets and towels, using disposable equipment or gowns, covering any sores, cuts, or other wounds, and disinfecting stethoscopes) is important for everyone in health care, including healers. Sometimes when healers clear "stuck" energy, they sense that it sticks to their hands. This feeling can be relieved by shaking the hands, washing them, holding them under cool running water, or touching the ground.

Q. *Can healers get exhausted by giving their energy to a patient?*

A. We've all had the experience of feeling tired after being around people who are depressed, anxious, or emotionally demanding, just as we've all felt energized after being with someone who is inspiring or charismatic. To avoid becoming personally depleted, healers should remember to remain centered and grounded. Avoid healing work when you are feeling tired or run down yourself; it is very difficult to remain centered and grounded in such a state, and it is much easier to become drained. It is helpful to visualize healing energy as flowing from an infinite, universal field of energy *through*, not *from*, the healer. Some types of Qigong healers extend their own vitality or energy to a recipient during treatment, and this can lead to fatigue. I recommend that you consider yourself a vehicle or channel instead. And remember, doing anything over a period of time can be tiring. Do take breaks, monitor yourself, and take care of yourself. You will not be helpful to others if you let yourself become run down.

Q. *My friend is pregnant. Should my treatments for her be twice as long now that she's eating for two?*

A. No. Healing sessions should be shorter and gentler for women who are pregnant, the very young, the elderly, those in shock, those who have suffered a head injury, and the extremely ill.

*Q. I've heard dermatologists say, "If it's dry, wet it; if it's wet, dry it."
Are there similar rules for healing?*

A. Yes. If it's agitated or painful, soothe it. If it's debilitated, energize it. If it's chaotic, organize it. If it's rigid, congested, or stuck, move it or empty it. If it's hot, cool it. If it's cold, warm it. If it's scattered and chaotic, restore harmony. If it's unbalanced, balance it. Hold to your own centered sense of peace, harmony, and well-being. Allow that inner sense of strength and stability to resonate through your words and actions.

Q. Should I keep records?

A. Yes. One of the best ways to learn is to document carefully what you sense, what you think, and what you did during a healing treatment. Comparing your experiences with different people over time will help you learn and keep you honest with yourself. Ask for feedback from recipients and others who care for them. Compare with colleagues who also offer healing treatments. Compare your impressions with standard diagnostic tests, imaging studies, and laboratory assessments.

Keeping written records has one cost (it takes time) and numerous benefits. The benefits include:

- Improved sensitivity to clues
- Greater insight
- Better collaboration
- Enhanced honesty and open-minded inquiry
- Reduced fantasies and self-delusions

Finally, written records may be required if you are offering services in a professional capacity or health care setting or if you are seeking formal certification in a specific technique like Therapeutic Touch or Healing Touch.

Q: What if I'm not sure what treatment to offer?

A: Uncertainty happens. It is always safe to focus yourself on being centered and grounded. If you are not certain what to do for someone else, you have a lot of options: ask what they want; ask for advice from someone else; refer them to a health professional; wait until you have clarity. It is much better to ask or refer than to act out of ignorance and delay appropriate help.

Q: What do you call the kind of healing work you offer?

A: For myself, I refer to it as Compassionate Healing Intention because I like the acronym (CHI). In general when I'm talking with colleagues, students, or patients, I try to describe what I'm doing in simple language that makes sense to them. When in doubt, describe exactly what you are doing: "touching gently while extending thoughts of kindness and healing"; "cradling the painful part in my hands while taking slow, relaxing breaths to help create a sense of ease and relaxation"; "sweeping my hands lightly over the body to soothe and comfort."

Q: Where can I get in-person training?

In North America, nursing organizations have been in the forefront of offering training in healing.

- The American Holistic Nurses Association
- Healing Touch International
- Nurse Healers Professional Associates International (Therapeutic Touch)

- Therapeutic Touch International Association

Trust your intuition. And seek sessions with different healers in your area. You may find a Reiki master or Qigong master who is willing to offer training, or a shaman or spiritual healer who offers healing ceremonies. Keep an open mind (but not so open your brains fall out). Just as there is no single flavor of ice cream that's everyone's favorite, there is not a single type or technique of healing work that's best for everyone. If you remain open, curious, and kind-hearted, you will find ways to be helpful and healing. Please let me know what you learn so I can learn from you.

CHAPTER 20
Resources

NOW THAT YOU'VE COVERED THE BASICS, are you ready for more? There is nothing like training with an expert in person. There are also wonderful books, organizations, and more resources for a lifetime of learning. Here is a sample of those that have been helpful to me.

Books on Healing: Overview

Chopra D., *The Path to Love: Spiritual Strategies for Healing*, (Harmony, 1998).

Chopra D., *Journey into Healing: Awakening the Wisdom Within You*, (Harmony, 1994).

Gerber R., *Vibrational Medicine: the #1 Handbook of Subtle-Energy Therapies*, (Bear and Company, 2001).

Gerber R., *A Practical Guide to Vibrational Medicine: Energy Healing and Spiritual Transformation*, (William Morrow Paperbacks, 2001).

Goswami A., *The Quantum Doctor: A Quantum Physicist Explains the Healing Power of Integral Medicine*, (Hampton Roads Publishing, 2011).

Hay L., *You can Heal Your Life*, (Hay House, 1984).

Jonas W.B. and Crawford C.C., *Healing, Intention, and Energy Medicine: Science, Research Methods and Clinical Implications*, (Churchill Livingstone, 2003).

LeShan L., *How to Meditate: A Guide to Self-Discovery*, (Little, Brown, and Company, 1999).

Loes M., *The Healing Response: How to Help Your Body Heal Itself*, (Freedom Press, Inc., 2004).

Shealy N., *Energy Medicine: Practical Applications and Scientific Proof*, (A.R.E. Press, 2011).

Weil A., *Spontaneous Healing: How to Discover and Embrace Your Body's Natural Ability to Maintain and Heal Itself* , (Ballantine Books, 2000).

Journals
Subtle Energies and Energy Medicine, International Society for the Study of Subtle Energies and Energy Medicine (ISSSEEM)

Books on Specific Kinds of Healing

Brennan School

Brennan B.A., *Hands of Light: A Guide to Healing Through the Human Energy Field*, (Bantam, 1988).

Brennan B.A., *Light Emerging: The Journey of Personal Healing*, (Bantam, 1993).

Bruyere Method

Bruyere R., *Wheels of Light: Chakras, Auras, and the Healing Energy of the Body*, (Touchstone, 1994).

Healing Touch

Hover-Kramer D., *Healing Touch: A Guidebook for Practitioners*, (Cengage Learning, 2001).

Hover-Kramer D., *Healing Touch: Essential Energy Medicine for Yourself and Others*, (Sounds True, 2011).

Polarity Therapy

Ross C.L., *Etiology: How to Detect Disease in Your Energy Field Before It Manifests in Your Body*, (XLibris, 2013).

Pranic Healing

Co S. and Robins E.B., *Your Hands Can Heal You: Pranic Healing Energy Remedies to Boost Vitality and Speed Recovery from Common Health Problems*, (Atria Books, 2004).

Prayer

Dossey L., *Healing Words: The Power of Prayer and the Practice of Medicine*, (HarperOne, 1995).

Dossey L., *Prayer is Good Medicine: How to Reap the Healing Benefits of Prayer*, (HarperOne, 1997).

Reiki

Miles P., *Reiki: A Comprehensive Guide*, (Tarcher, 2008).

Shamanism

Carson C. (editor), *Spirited Medicine: Shamanism in Contemporary Healthcare*, (Otter Bay Books, 2013).

Therapeutic Touch

Krieger D., *The Therapeutic Touch: How to Use Your Hands to Help or to Heal*, (Touchstone, 1979).

Krieger D., *Accepting Your Power to Heal: the Personal Practice of Therapeutic Touch*, (Santa Fe: Bear and Company, 1993).

Krieger D., *Therapeutic Touch: Inner Workbook*, (Bear and Company, 1997).

Krieger D., *Therapeutic Touch as Transpersonal Healing*, (New York: Lantern/BookLight, 2002).

Kunz D., and Krieger D., *The Spiritual Dimension of Therapeutic Touch*, (Bear and Company, 2004).

MacRae J., *Therapeutic Touch: A Practical Guide*, (Alfred A Knopf, 1988).

May D., *Therapeutic Touch Handbook: Level Basic*, (Scribe Press, 2001).

May D., *Therapeutic Touch Handbooks, Levels 2 & 3: Intermediate*, (Scribe Press, 2003).

May D., *Therapeutic Touch Handbook: Advanced Practice*, (Scribe Press, 2013).

Wager S., *Doctor's Guide to Therapeutic Touch: Enhancing the Body's Energy to Promote Healing*, (Perigee Books, 1996).

Index

Kunz, Dora, 16, 18, 31, 44, 50, 122, 169, 274, 283

L
Lacteal ducts, 150
Lamashtu Healers, 44
Lamott, Anne, 134
Large Intestine 4 (LI4), 163–164
Large intestine (yang) meridian, 163
Larrimore, Deborah, 267
Laying on of hands, 60
Laziness, guarding against, 69
Leadbetter, C. W., 169
Liver 3 (Lv3), 164
Liver (yin) meridian, 162
Loving-kindness, 106
  defined, 109
  extending, 111–112
  related to self-compassion, 110
Low Dog, Tieraona, 81
Lumbosacral plexus, 153
Lung (yin) meridian, 163
Lungs, 148
Lymphatic system, anatomy of, 150–151
Lymph nodes, 150

M
Marma points, 157
McCraty, Rollin, 149
McGarey, Gladys, 273–274
Medical Qigong, 57
Meditation
  benefits of, and brain structure, 115
  centering as form of, 34
  concentration-based (focused-attention), 113, 114–116
  insight meditation, 116–120
  mindfulness, 113, 116–120
  origin of word, 113
  sitting meditation, 118–119
  types of, 113–114
  walking meditation, 119
Mental body, 292
  characteristics of, 169

Mental health, Therapeutic Touch and, 52
Mental preparation
  biofeedback, 129–130
  concentration-based meditation, 114–116
  guided imagery, 120–126
  journaling, 128–129
  mindfulness, 116–120
  summary of, 130–131
Mentgen, Janet, 44, 53
Meridians
  location and active time, 161–163
  meridian pairs, 161–163
  overview, 160–161
  yin and yang meridians, 161–163
Metronome, 83
Mind-Body Medicine, Center for, 121
Mindfulness
  attention, 118
  attitude, 117–118
  body scan, 118
  defined, 97, 113
  intention, 117
  keys to, 117–118
  movement and, 119–120
  overview of, 116–117
  sitting meditation, 118–119
Mindfulness in Medicine, Health Care, Center for, 117
Mineral anatomy, 169
Modern medicine anatomy, 147–156
  cardiovascular system, 148–149
  endocrine system, 154
  lymphatic system, 150–151
  musculo-skeletal and connective tissue system, 154–155
  nervous system, 151–154
  skin, 155–156
Motivations for becoming healer, 23–28
Moving high to low vs. low to high; moving inward vs. outward warm-up exercise, 188–190
Muscles, healing and, 154–155

About the Author

DR. KATHI J. KEMPER, M.D., M.P.H., received her medical and public health training at the University of North Carolina and her pediatric specialty training at the University of Wisconsin. She has served on the faculty of Yale University, University of Washington, Wake Forest University, Harvard Medical School, and the Ohio State University. Dr. Kemper served as the founding director of centers for integrative medicine at Boston Children's Hospital, Wake Forest, and Ohio State. She is Past President of the Academic Pediatric Association and founded the American Academy of Pediatrics' Section on Integrative Medicine. Her work has been published in leading medical journals, including the *New England Journal of Medicine*, the *Journal of the American Medical Association,* and *Academic Medicine*. Her pioneering work in integrative medicine and mentoring women has been recognized with numerous awards, including the Library of Congress's "Women Who Dare." Dr. Kemper is recognized internationally as the leading authority on complementary therapies for children, and she is frequently consulted by media, including *The New York Times, Chicago Tribune, Newsweek,* ABC News, *The Wall Street Journal, Reader's Digest, Redbook, First for Women,* and *USA Today.* She has published over 160 peer-reviewed research papers and three other books for the public *(The Holistic Pediatrician; Mental Health, Naturally; Addressing ADD Naturally).* She is the happy mother of a wonderful son, Daniel, and a faithful servant to three cats. She enjoys gardening, music, hiking in the mountains, strolling by the sea, and helping kindred spirits connect, grow, and contribute together to improve lives.